D0012129

*Praise for*
## The Procrastinator's Guide to Getting Things Done

"Do you hold off to the last minute on those less-than-pleasant tasks? Are you typically off by 50% on your 'that-won't-take-long-I've-got-time' estimates? Think you are a capital-P Procrastinator for life? With this guide, you'll get the quick-and-easy shortcuts around all your excuses. You'll gain the tools to find your personal stall tactics and the repair kit to fix them. When you're done, get ready for your reward: efficient productivity and more time for fun."
—*Reid Wilson, PhD, author of* Don't Panic

"Filled with examples of people who have overcome procrastination, practical and powerful advice, and helpful forms, this book can help you change your life. Read it and use it—what are you waiting for?"
—*Robert L. Leahy, PhD, author of* The Worry Cure

"Turns out it *does* take one to know one! As a procrastinator of many years, I found observations and examples I could relate to in every chapter. Dr. Basco will help you understand why you keep procrastinating, even though it does more harm than good—and how to beat it once and for all."
—*Eric A., lawyer*

"This book is a treasure trove of practical methods to break procrastinating habits. Dr. Basco will inspire you and cheer you on as you learn how to become a 'doer.' I wish this book had been available sooner. It would have saved me many hours and days of spinning my wheels."
—*Jesse H. Wright, MD, PhD, Department of Psychiatry and Behavioral Sciences; Director, Depression Center; and Vice Chair for Academic Affairs, University of Louisville*

"I thought I had my self-defeating procrastination habits under control, but when I saw myself in so many of this book's scenarios, I realized I still have work to do. Fortunately, Dr. Basco provides simple steps to move from overwhelmed to active; from stalling to success. I gained new insights, great reminders, and thoughtful encouragement—all of which have helped me to shift the way I approach tasks and safeguard against falling into the same old traps."
—*Susan L. Franzen, Director, Leadership Institute, University of Texas System*

# The Procrastinator's Guide to Getting Things Done

# The Procrastinator's Guide to
# Getting Things Done

Monica Ramirez Basco, PhD

THE GUILFORD PRESS
New York    London

© 2010 The Guilford Press
A Division of Guilford Publications, Inc.
72 Spring Street, New York, NY 10012
www.guilford.com

All rights reserved

The information in this volume is not intended as a substitute for
consultation with healthcare professionals. Each individual's health
concerns should be evaluated by a qualified professional.

Except as indicated, no part of this book may be reproduced,
translated, stored in a retrieval system, or transmitted, in any
form or by any means, electronic, mechanical, photocopying,
microfilming, recording, or otherwise, without written permission
from the publisher.

Printed in the United States of America

This book is printed on acid-free paper.

Last digit is print number:  9  8  7  6  5  4  3  2  1

LIMITED PHOTOCOPY LICENSE

The publisher grants to individual purchasers of this book
nonassignable permission to reproduce pages 9–11 of this
book. This license is limited to you, the individual purchaser,
for personal use or use with individual clients. This license
does not grant the right to reproduce these materials for
resale, redistribution, electronic display, or any other purposes
(including but not limited to books, pamphlets, articles, video-
or audiotapes, blogs, file-sharing sites, Internet or intranet sites,
and handouts or slides for lectures, workshops, webinars, or
therapy groups, whether or not a fee is charged). Permission to
reproduce these materials for these and any other purposes must
be obtained in writing from the Permissions Department of
Guilford Publications.

Library of Congress Cataloging-in-Publication Data

Basco, Monica Ramirez.
    The procrastinator's guide to getting things done /
Monica Ramirez Basco.
       p.     cm.
    Includes index.
    ISBN 978-1-60623-293-4 (pbk. : alk. paper)
    ISBN 978-1-60623-462-4 (hardcover : alk. paper)
    1. Procrastination.   2. Self-actualization (Psychology)
I. Title.
    BF637.P76B37 2010
    155.2′32—dc22
                                                    2009033268

# Contents

# Preface

I have been procrastinating on starting this book for some time now. I told myself I would get to it later, when I was in a more creative mood, but that mood still hasn't occurred. I told myself I would get to it as soon as I finished a few other pressing tasks, but those tasks are still not done. I told myself I would start working on it as soon as my summer break from classes started. Classes ended four weeks ago. I even told myself I would start working on it tomorrow. That was two weeks ago. This sounds like procrastination to me.

I know it must seem odd that someone writing a book on how to stop procrastinating is as stuck as her readers. People are always surprised to hear that I procrastinate, because I always seem busy. In fact, I always *am* busy. I have been married for 30 years, raised three sons, been a college professor for 22 years, treated many people in my clinical practice, and managed to write a few books, scrub many toilets, wash truckloads of dishes, and cook more meals than I can count, and I've had a lot of fun in the process. I don't look like a procrastinator on the surface, but what I know about myself is that there have been plenty of times when I have waited until the last minute to get things done, done more enjoyable tasks instead of the less enjoyable ones, or put off things that were too hard to do. I have delayed starting unpleasant tasks. I have told myself that tomorrow would be a better day to start a project even when that wasn't true. And I have scrambled to meet a deadline when I could have started sooner and not put myself into a panic. The reason people do not think I am a procrastinator is that while I was delaying, or putting things off, or waiting until the last minute to start a task, I was not just sitting around. I was doing one of a thousand other things that were on my to-do list. Although I could easily justify my choices and my actions, I knew in each of these cases that I was procrastinating on something I didn't really want to do.

There are many kinds of procrastinators. I am not the blissful type. I can't procrastinate and just relax and do nothing. Even when I decide to put something off for a while, my brain sends out periodic reminders that things need to be done. It is really quite annoying. I am not able to enjoy the peace and quiet that procrastination is supposed to provide. The whole idea behind procrastination is that you can at least temporarily free yourself of worry about a task until you are ready to get to it.

As it turns out, many procrastinators are just like me. They may decide to put off what they are not in the mood to deal with at present, but they can't really shake it from their minds. Procrastination makes them feel bad, guilty, worried, overwhelmed, and stressed. They know that if they just got things done, they would not have to feel bad about not getting things done. Although that reasoning seems perfectly logical, it does not help them take action. In fact, most procrastinators realize what they are doing and know they have to take action to make it stop, but they feel powerless to change. They ask themselves, "Why am I like this?" but they never get a straight answer. They think if they could figure out why they procrastinate, they would stop doing it.

The purpose of this book is to do just that, to help you figure out why you procrastinate and what to do about it. While the book is organized to help with both gaining understanding and taking action, you need to know that fixing the problem of procrastination does not require you to fully understand why you do it. In fact, you can gain a full understanding of how you came to be a procrastinator, why you do it, and what keeps it going and still not change your behavior. Some of you will find that learning more about what is behind your procrastination might be enough to make quick changes. For others, the process may take more time and effort even if you understand what makes you tick. If you are in the second group, patience and persistence will be needed but should pay off in the long run.

You will also learn that the label *procrastinator* is a negative one that only serves to make the problem worse. It implies that procrastination is a character trait that can't be changed. An important thesis of this book is that procrastination is a behavior and that behaviors can be improved. Through exercises, examples, and instructions, you can learn to control your tendency to avoid, delay, or put things off.

There are many different reasons that people get tripped up by procrastination. Some people worry about their ability to do things right. When faced with something new or challenging, their anxiety or self-doubt makes them put things off until the last possible minute. Some people delay on tasks they don't want to do. There always seems to something much more fun or interesting to do first. By comparison, things they "have to do" seem unpleasant. Some people delay because they are not well organized and can't figure out where to start. Some people delay because they doubt themselves and their ability to complete a task or project. Some use procrastination as a way of making a point to others that they will not be told what to do. You may have encountered one or all of these roadblocks on your life path.

It is hard to stop procrastinating, because it usually works. Most procrastinators find a way to get things done. It may be at the last minute, the end result may be not as good as they would have liked, it may be a little late, and sometimes there is a penalty for its tardiness, but one way or another it usually gets done. You know this well. You are probably reading this book because you are tired of procrastinating. You know that it is a habit you could potentially keep for the rest of your life, but you want to change.

You can learn to do things differently. You do not have to continue down the path of procrastination. If you are like most procrastinators, you probably just don't know a different way. To help get you on the right track, the first chapter provides you with an opportunity to take a procrastination test. It will help you figure out what might be driving your procrastination. When you add up your score, you will figure out what type of procrastination describes you best. You can use this information to zero in on the chapters that will best meet your needs. The second chapter will start you off on the right foot by providing a number of *Shortcuts*. They won't resolve procrastination altogether, but they will give you some quick fixes that can help you gain confidence in your ability to overcome your procrastination. Throughout the book, you will find additional Shortcuts and sections called *Changing Directions* where you will learn new ways to cope. These more advanced skills will help you in a variety of situations, and if you practice them you can make some permanent changes in your procrastination. Chapters 3–8 each cover a different type of procrastination. The Shortcuts and Changing Directions exercises in these chapters are designed specifically for those types. You can read the book from cover to cover, or you can skip to the chapters that you think will be most applicable to you. Most people who procrastinate do so for a variety of reasons, depending on the situation and the task. Therefore, you might find it helpful to read all of the chapters. In fact, since the chapters build on each other, you might find that you get more out of them if you do read them in order.

This book approaches procrastination from a perspective called *cognitive-behavioral therapy*, or CBT. It is a type of psychotherapy that has been proven effective in the treatment of a variety of disorders such as depression and anxiety, as well as stress, chronic pain, and relationship problems. My expertise is in this area of treatment, and I have been involved in research and teaching in CBT for most of my career. I like CBT methods because they have been well tested and they are fairly easy to teach. I do a lot of training of students and professional therapists in CBT for depression, anxiety, and bipolar disorder. Trainees find CBT easy to learn and can then pass on these strategies to the people they treat. Throughout this book, you will learn many of the same methods that I teach therapists-in-training and that I teach my patients.

As I look back on my procrastination in starting this book, I have to say that I never quite figured out why I was putting it off. Now that I am writing I know that it feels pretty good, like a small weight has been lifted from my shoulders. It might have been that I didn't know where to start. Maybe it was because I lacked confidence in my ability to write it. Or maybe I was just lazy. Any or all of these obstacles might have blocked my progress, but for now it doesn't seem to matter. I hope that by taking action myself I can help you take action.

# The Procrastinator's Guide to Getting Things Done

# 1  Why Do I Procrastinate?

**Directions:**

| | |
|---|---|
| START: | Find out why people procrastinate. |
| ⟹ | Admit that procrastination works for you. |
| ⟹ | Measure the severity of your problem. |
| ⟹ | Learn to recognize the urge to procrastinate. |
| END: | Commit to making a change. |

There is a good chance that you are reading this book because you are unhappy with yourself. You have probably been procrastinating on things for some time, have tried to change on your own, and have not been very successful. If you are like most procrastinators, you have probably made promises to yourself that the next time you are faced with a task you will not wait until the last minute to get it done. In fact, you have probably made that promise more than once and have had trouble keeping it. This book is for people who:

- Don't understand why they procrastinate.
- Feel bad about doing it.
- Wish that they didn't.
- Want to change, but don't know how.

Procrastination is hard to change. It is not something you can just decide to give up and then completely let it go. It is a well-worn path in your life, a habit that is so automatic that it does not require thought or planning. It is not like you open your eyes in the morning and say, "I think I'm going to procrastinate today." It is actually quite the opposite. You start your day saying that you will not take that path, fall into that habit, and yet without realizing it you find yourself there again. Procrastination might be that slight pause where you intend to do a task but hesitate and then turn away. Maybe you reach for the phone to call someone and then change your mind and tell yourself that you will do it later. Or you go to the kitchen with the intention of washing the dishes, you see the mess, and then you leave the room to do something else. Procrastination occurs when you start a task like paying your bills and then find yourself cleaning out a drawer instead. It's also those times when you find yourself spending more time getting ready to do a task, like straightening up your office before you work, than actually doing the work. It is like driving down the road toward your destination and then turning off in another direction at the last moment.

Procrastination is our comfort zone. It is where we feel the most at ease. It is familiar. We know how to do it. It doesn't challenge us or scare us. Procrastination gives us temporary comfort in a world full of demands and uncertainties. It is our rest stop on the long road of life and responsibilities.

Procrastination is also an altered state of reality. It is our happy place. It allows us to believe temporarily that we have nothing to do. It pushes our to-do list so far out of our minds that for a short while we can almost believe the list does not exist. It makes us believe we deserve to rest, relax, and take it easy. It makes us feel bold in justifying our inaction, inactivity, hesitation, and avoidance.

Procrastination is a roadblock on your life path. It slows your progress and sometimes takes you off course altogether.

Procrastination is seductive. It allows you to have a little bit of joy or pleasure or relief from stress. It takes away the things you hate to do and replaces them with something better. It keeps you from having to deal with unpleasant people and difficult chores. It allows you to delay getting bad news. It gives you five more minutes in the comfort of your bed on a cold winter morning.

Procrastination is, however, only a disguise. It masks your true thoughts and feelings. It masquerades as laziness, but it is much more than that. On the surface, procrastination looks like a comfortable, relaxing experience, but underneath it is full of guilt and self-loathing. Peacefulness is what we pretend to feel while we are procrastinating, yet it is anything but peaceful. While we are procrastinating we are watching ourselves do it. We are criticizing the behavior. We are filled with guilt for putting things off. We dread what will happen if we wait any longer to get started. We hate ourselves for doing it and call ourselves names such as "lazy," "irresponsible," "uncaring," "stupid," and "worthless." We act like we are relieved not to have to deal with whatever we are trying to ignore, but we are stressing on the inside, worrying about what we will eventually have to face. You have probably had experiences where you sat in front of the TV to watch the news for a few moments before getting started on your chores but were distracted by thoughts of what you needed to do next, so you missed what the announcer had to say. Or maybe for those extra few minutes you stayed in bed after turning off the alarm you lay there physically resting but mentally running through your list of responsibilities for the day. During these times we know that by procrastinating we are probably making it worse. That makes us anxious and also robs us of the desire to take action.

The *number one* reason that we procrastinate is BECAUSE WE CAN. The majority of the time things still get done and no real consequence is suffered. We get away with it when we are students by cramming at the last minute. We get away with it as adults by changing our minds and deciding not to do the task after all. We get away with it at work when another member of the team gets worried and picks up the slack. We get away with it at home because we can work around chores that are not finished or count on someone else doing them for us. We may suffer consequences, but they are usually not substantial. We get a late fee on our credit card bill or on our rent for not sending a payment in on time. So what? We pay it and manage without the extra money.

We live in a world of extra chances. The IRS will give us an extension when our taxes are not done on time. There are grace periods that allow us to delay without penalty. If we lose an opportunity, we can often find another one. We get warnings that we are approaching a deadline. We get alerts when we are about to run out of time, or power in our batteries, or minutes on our cell phones. For many everyday things we can afford to put things off a little, take our time, sit on it for a while, or sleep on it. Our modern world is full of opportunities to procrastinate.

How many times have you waited until the last minute but still gotten things done? How many extensions have you needed? How many apologies have you given for being late? How many late fees have you paid? You are probably aware of the many tasks you have consciously avoided because you just didn't feel like doing them, but how many more do you think you unconsciously avoided? Consider all these times when either nothing bad happened or the consequence was small and not a big deal. You were able to get away with it.

The big question is why we would want to give it up. Why do we feel guilty about it? Why do we pledge time and time again to change our ways? The reason may be that procrastination works only in the short run. It provides only temporary relief. In the long run, it does not get us where we want to go. We feel angry at ourselves for it when we step back and see the stress that it causes and how it interferes with our lives. If we could hold on to the big picture and see clearly where we want to go in life, we would choose not to procrastinate. If we could remember how much trouble it causes, we probably wouldn't procrastinate the next time. The problem is that we are so used to using procrastination as our coping strategy that we do it automatically, without considering the big picture. In the moment, when faced with something unpleasant, we just want to detour around it, and so we avoid, delay, put off, forget about, and otherwise procrastinate on it.

Procrastination is a common behavior. Some do it more than others. This book probably caught your attention because, just like me, you are not a blissful procrastinator. You want to change. That desire makes all the difference.

## ☙ *A Personal Note*

*Like everyone else, I don't like doing tasks that are unpleasant or stressful. There are some things I would like to avoid forever, but that is usually not possible in my world. I don't like that feeling of hesitation where my mind does a quick tug of war with my emotions: "You should do that now." "No, I don't want to!" I feel my gut tightening and a pressure in my chest. My upbringing leads me to feel a sensation of guilt while this is happening. Sometimes the guilt for thinking about putting something off is more unpleasant than the dread of doing the task. It's better if I just do the thing that I am avoiding and get it over with. My goal is to stop the tug of war and either put off a task intentionally, with good reason, and enjoy my moment of relief or just get up and take care of the task that is nagging at me.*

*What is your goal?*

## Procrastination Is a Way to Cope

If you are like most people, you probably associate procrastination with laziness. That is most likely because your parents or teachers told you to stop being lazy whenever they saw you put your work aside to relax, have some fun, watch TV, goof off, spend time on the computer, talk to your friends, or do anything else they thought was a waste of time. I remember teachers saying things like "Never put off till tomorrow what you can do today" or "Don't dilly-dally" or "You have to get your work done before you can go out and play." My mom had a few colorful words in Spanish for laziness that I would hear when I was parked in front of the television instead of doing my chores.

What I have come to learn through my personal experience as a mom, a psychologist, and a college professor is that there is much more to procrastination than laziness. Behind most procrastination is a task or activity that the person would like to get out of doing if he or she could. Often it is something that the person believes will be hard to do, unpleasant, or even painful in some way. Just the thought of it stirs up uncomfortable feelings like anxiety, dread, or anger. Procrastination is a way of shutting down those bad feelings. In this way, it is a type of self-preservation, a way to cope.

## ༀ A Personal Note

*I teach college students in the Psychology Department at the University of Texas at Arlington. It is a great deal of fun for me, and my students seem to enjoy my classes as well. I am one of those professors, however, who make their students write papers as part of their course requirements, and I never accept late papers unless there is a verifiable medical emergency. When I first began to do this, I got lots of calls from students within the last few days before the assignment was due, asking about the instructions for the paper. Clearly they had waited until the last minute, and most of the time their papers ended up showing a lack of preparation. My students are quite intelligent, so their poor performance was not due to lack of brainpower. It was due to procrastinating and running out of time.*

*In subsequent semesters I took time to ask students early in the semester if they were having trouble getting started on their papers. Many had not started and had no idea how to begin. Several voiced fear that they would "do it wrong" and were stuck in their fear. Some were busy having fun and told themselves that they had all the time in the world and were not at all worried about it.*

*They should have been worried. What they showed me is that procrastination is not laziness or irresponsibility. It is the way my students coped with their fear of making a mistake, their uncertainty and lack of self-confidence about the task, and it was a product of their false belief that they write better under pressure. Knowing this helps me address their concerns before the final paper is due. While we talk about the paper in class, I make them anxious because I force them to think about what they have been avoiding. For a while, I take away their ability to use procrastination as a way to cope. In the long run, however, they are pleased to have their questions answered and get their fears off their chest.*

Read through Changing Directions 1 to determine whether you are using procrastination as a coping strategy.

---

↺ Changing Directions 1

## Are You Using Procrastination as a Way to Cope?

Read each question and put a check next to the ones to which you would answer yes.

- ❏ If you feel uncertain, will you postpone taking action or making a decision?

- ❏ When you are mentally or physically tired, do you tell yourself you will do it later?

- ❏ If you dread having to face a problem or a difficult person, will you avoid it for as long as you can?

- ❏ If you are nervous about having to do something difficult, will you delay?

- ❏ If you are angry about being forced to do something you don't want to do, will you procrastinate?

- ❏ If you are afraid you are going to make a mistake or mess things up, do you wait too long to start a task?

- ❏ If you have to face a person who is unpleasant, will you make an excuse to put it off?

If you answered yes to any of these questions, you are using procrastination as a way to cope.

---

## How Bad Is It?

Procrastination is a common behavior, and doing it once in a while doesn't usually cause problems. Most of the time you are the only person who suffers. At least that is what you tell yourself. Your first step toward overcoming procrastination is to be honest with yourself about how often it happens and how much trouble it is causing you. Try Changing Directions 2. See if you really are the world's worst procrastinator or just a normal everyday procrastinator.

---

↺ Changing Directions 2
**Procrastination Quiz**

For each item, rate the extent to which the problems with procrastination occur in your personal life, at school, at work, and at home. Be honest with yourself. For each item, indicate how often it occurs. Use the following scale.

0 = **It never happens.**

1 = **It happens sometimes.**

2 = **It happens fairly often.**

3 = **It happens a lot more often than I would like.**

Add up your score for each subscale. Think about whether the behaviors in each subscale are more of a problem at work, in your home life, at school, in your relationships with others, or just in personal matters that affect you and not necessarily other people. Check the domain at the bottom of the subscale that applies most. It is OK to pick more than one.

You will tally up the subscales at the end of the quiz to determine the severity of your problem with procrastination.

---

| Subscale 1 | How often does this happen? |
|---|---|
| 1. I put things off, and they don't get done. | |
| 2. While I procrastinate, I still keep thinking about what I should be doing. | |
| 3. Other people are on my case for procrastinating. | |
| 4. My procrastination makes me late for lots of things. | |
| 5. I make excuses for not getting started. | |
| SUBSCALE 1 | |
| Where do you have the most trouble with this? (✓) | |
| ( ) Work    ( ) Home    ( ) School    ( ) Relationship    ( ) Self | |

| Subscale 2 | How often does this happen? |
|---|---|
| 6. I avoid stressful situations and tasks. | |
| 7. When a task stresses me out, I wait until the last minute to do it. | |
| 8. I ignore unpleasant tasks until the last minute. | |
| 9. I avoid bad news. | |
| 10. I avoid information I don't really want to hear. | |
| SUBSCALE 2 | |
| Where do you have the most trouble with this? (✓) | |
| ( ) Work    ( ) Home    ( ) School    ( ) Relationship    ( ) Self | |

| Subscale 3 | How often does this happen? |
|---|---|
| 11. I tell myself I have plenty of time even when that's not true. | |

From *The Procrastinator's Guide to Getting Things Done* by Monica Ramirez Basco. Copyright 2010 by The Guilford Press.

| | |
|---|---|
| 12. I have trouble getting organized. | |
| 13. I underestimate how long it will take to get things done. | |
| 14. I overestimate how much time I have available to get things done. | |
| 15. I put off tasks because I can't concentrate. | |
| **SUBSCALE 3** | |
| Where do you have the most trouble with this? (✓) | |
| ( ) Work    ( ) Home    ( ) School    ( ) Relationship    ( ) Self | |

| Subscale 4 | How often does this happen? |
|---|---|
| 16. I hesitate because I am afraid of making a mistake or failing. | |
| 17. I avoid taking actions that others might not like. | |
| 18. I avoid things that I am unsure about. | |
| 19. My self-doubt and uncertainty make me postpone getting started on difficult tasks. | |
| 20. I am not always sure what decision to make, so I put it off as long as possible. | |
| **SUBSCALE 4** | |
| Where do you have the most trouble with this? (✓) | |
| ( ) Work    ( ) Home    ( ) School    ( ) Relationship    ( ) Self | |

| Subscale 5 | How often does this happen? |
|---|---|
| 21. I hate being told what to do. | |
| 22. I intentionally procrastinate when others tell me what to do. | |
| 23. I show my displeasure by stalling. | |

From *The Procrastinator's Guide to Getting Things Done* by Monica Ramirez Basco. Copyright 2010 by The Guilford Press.

| | |
|---|---|
| 24. I agree to do things for others that I later regret. | |
| 25. It's hard for me to say no to people. | |
| SUBSCALE 5 | |

Where do you have the most trouble with this? (✓)
( ) Work ( ) Home ( ) School ( ) Relationship ( ) Self

| Subscale 6 | How often does this happen? |
|---|---|
| 26. I take on more than I can handle. | |
| 27. If I can't do something perfectly, I won't do it at all. | |
| 28. I get overwhelmed by too much to do. | |
| 29. I either give my all or put things off altogether. | |
| 30. I work so hard at times that I wear myself out. | |
| SUBSCALE 6 | |

Where do you have the most trouble with this? (✓)
( ) Work ( ) Home ( ) School ( ) Relationship ( ) Self

| Subscale 7 | How often does this happen? |
|---|---|
| 31. I play instead of work. | |
| 32. When I don't feel motivated, I don't take action. | |
| 33. It's hard for me to stop doing something fun or relaxing and get back to tasks. | |
| 34. I avoid unpleasant tasks until someone does them for me. | |
| 35. I have no real excuse for procrastinating. | |
| SUBSCALE 7 | |

Where do you have the most trouble with this? (✓)
( ) Work ( ) Home ( ) School ( ) Relationship ( ) Self

From *The Procrastinator's Guide to Getting Things Done* by Monica Ramirez Basco. Copyright 2010 by The Guilford Press.

Add up your subscale scores in the following table. Next to each subscale is a description of the type of procrastinator you might be. Read on to learn more about these subtypes.

| | |
|---|---|
| Subscale 1—General Characteristics | |
| Subscale 2—Avoidant Type | |
| Subscale 3—Disorganized Type | |
| Subscale 4—Self-Doubting Type | |
| Subscale 5—Interpersonal Type | |
| Subscale 6—All-or-Nothing Type | |
| Subscale 7—Pleasure-Seeking Type | |
| **GRAND TOTAL** | |

## How Bad Is It?

- 0 to 35 = **Normal**. Don't worry about it. You don't procrastinate enough for it to be a problem.

- 36 to 60 = **Mild**. You still manage to get things done, but the stress is getting to you. You know you could do so much better if you didn't procrastinate.

- 61 to 70 = **Moderate**. Your procrastination is a problem. Not only do you know that you procrastinate, but the people who know you also know you are a procrastinator. This is embarrassing for you.

- 71 to 105 = **Severe**. It's time to make some serious changes.

# What Type of Procrastinator Are You?

There are six types of procrastinators, each with a unique reason for putting things off. Each of the Procrastination Quiz subscales relates to a different type. Items 1 through 5 are general problems with procrastination that are common to all types of procrastinators such as Bob. Bob knows he puts things off when he shouldn't, and he feels guilty about it. When he was married, his wife got on his case about it, especially when his delays made them both late for appointments.

Items 6 through 10 are rated highly by avoiders. Avoiders cope with stress and unpleasantness by putting things off as long as possible. Donna has to tell her grandmother that she is getting a divorce. Donna knows her grandmother will not approve of this because no one in her family has ever been divorced. The conversation is going to be very stressful, so Donna keeps putting it off.

Items 11 to 15 are typically checked by the disorganized type of procrastinator. People in this group underestimate how long tasks can take and overestimate how much time they have available. They have trouble setting priorities when there is too much to do. Freddie, for example, wastes time on small tasks as a way of avoiding bigger ones; he will, for example, reorganize his CDs instead of cleaning his room.

Items 16 through 20 pertain to procrastinators who are self-doubters. They hesitate to take action because they lack confidence in their abilities. They think they will make a mistake or fail. Arthur, for example, isn't sure how to put together the end-of-year budget summary for his procrastination support group. He puts off doing it because he is afraid it won't be right.

Items 21 through 25 pertain to the interpersonal type of procrastinator. These people procrastinate intentionally as a way of making a point. For example, Carla hates being told what to do, especially by someone at work who is not her boss. She always gets things done on time, but she stalls in getting started just to make people nervous that the job won't get done.

Items 26 to 30 relate to all-or-nothing procrastination. These are people who take on too much and work at full speed until they run out of steam. They can be binge workers who try to do it all until they get overwhelmed and shut down altogether. Olivia is an example of an all-or-nothing procrastinator. She agrees to help out on too many things and then gets completely overwhelmed by how much she has to do and how little time she has to do it all, so she shuts down and does nothing.

Items 31 through 35 fall into the pleasure-seeking subtype. Evelyn, for example, watches TV instead of typing up her report for class even though she knows she has a deadline and is running out of time. People who fall into this category sometimes call themselves "lazy" or "unmotivated."

## How to Use This Book

The rest of the chapters in this book are organized around these various subtypes of procrastinators. You might be tempted to use the subscale scores as a guide and skip to the section that pertains to the reasons you procrastinate. That's fine if it seems like the best way to get yourself going. But if your overall score is in the moderate or severe range, you probably procrastinate for a lot of different reasons, meaning several chapters may pertain to your kind of procrastination. To get the most out of this book, I recommend that you work through the chapters from beginning to end and perhaps use only the exercises that pertain to your specific problem. Keep in mind that the exercises presented throughout the book might pertain to more than one type of procrastination.

Another reason to consider reading this book from cover to cover is that the people just introduced are discussed throughout the chapters. You will learn more about them as you go through the examples, with each building on the characters' stories.

A strategy you might use as you work your way through this book is to focus on the area of your life where procrastination is causing you the most trouble. Review the domains you checked off at the bottom of each subscale. Is there a pattern of procrastinating more at work than in your personal life? Is it a bigger problem at school? Pick the area of your life where you may be procrastinating the most or where your problem is the most severe. Focus your energy on fixing the type of procrastination that occurs in that trouble spot. Or do what some people find gets them started and begin with the area that is easiest to improve on. Once you feel more confident in your ability to steer clear of procrastination, you can take on new life domains. Examples of how to address procrastination at work, school, and home, and in your personal life are provided in each chapter. You will pick up clues to coping as you read along.

The exercises that are presented start simple and build in complexity. If you can master some of the basic skills presented in the first few chapters, you will be more prepared to take on bigger changes as you read on.

## You Are Not Alone

When people are at the crossroads of procrastination or action, they pause there thinking about what they should do and how much they don't want to do it. They assume they are alone at that juncture because everyone else seems to be on top of things. This could not be further from the truth. If you don't believe it, ask ten people you know if they ever procrastinate. Then ask them if they wish they didn't. You are in good company.

### Procrastinators Support Group Chapter 121

Evelyn, Donna, Arthur, Carla, Bob, Freddie, Olivia, and others are members of Chapter 121 of the Procrastinators Support Group. They found each other through an online chat room for procrastinators. When they figured out that they did not live far from one another, they decided to meet in person. They have been meeting weekly in the back room of a diner off Highway 121. Donna, Arthur, Bob, and Evelyn are the longest-standing members and have become friends. Others have joined and left the group over the years. As mentioned, you will hear the group members' stories and read about their struggles throughout this book. If you have similar stories, you might find that their solutions to procrastination work for you too.

## Recognize the Urge to Procrastinate

Review your answers to the Procrastination Quiz. Each example of procrastination provides you with an opportunity for improvement. The items you rated as happening "fairly often" or "a lot more often than I would like" (2 or 3) can be used to help you recognize the warning signs that procrastination could occur since that's where you are currently procrastinating most. These warning signs place you at a fork in the road: when you see one, you can consciously decide to take action or procrastinate rather than falling automatically into old habits. Let's say you know you really hate it when people try to tell you what do to (high scores in subscale 5). Then, when your boss cavalierly hands you some extra work without asking if you have time or your brother assumes you'll take your mother to the doctor without asking if you'd mind, you'll be reminded that you are probably going to procrastinate just to resist being controlled. Another example is worry. If you know that worry makes you procrastinate on something you dread, the feeling of worry can be your cue that you are likely to cope by procrastinating.

The more aware you are that procrastination is about to occur, the better your chances of taking a different path and avoiding that roadblock. Self-awareness gives you control. There is a big difference between unconsciously procrastinating and doing it on purpose. Arthur wasn't always aware that fear of making a mistake was causing him to procrastinate. He just thought he was being lazy. Once he learned that self-doubt was his problem, he could decide to cope with stressful situations by putting things off or by finding another way to cope with his lack of confidence. Bob was the same way. Once he figured out that he was using procrastination as a way to communicate his anger to his ex-wife, he could consciously make the decision to speak up for himself rather than coping in a more passive way. Self-awareness gave them more choices and therefore more control.

Keep in mind as you make your way through the exercises in this book that procrastination is a choice. Sometimes it will be a reasonable choice, depending on the situation. When you have control over it, you can choose to procrastinate when the time is right, and you can choose how long to let it go on. Donna, for example, was having a very difficult time dealing with the fact that her marriage of 10 years was coming to an end. She knew that she had to tell her grandmother, a devout Catholic, about it and that based on her religious beliefs she would protest and try to talk Donna out of it. Donna was ambivalent about her decision to file for divorce and knew that if her grandmother pushed her on it, she might give in and call it off. Donna procrastinated in telling her grandmother about the divorce because she thought it was best to avoid her grandmother's wrath until she was feeling emotionally strong enough to stand her ground and cope with her grandmother's disapproval. Donna knew that her grandmother would eventually find out about the divorce and she could avoid the subject until someone else broke the bad news to her. Knowing this gave her control over the decision of whether to avoid her grandmother and how long to procrastinate in talking with her.

## Commit to Change

Everyone procrastinates some of the time. The goal is not to eliminate the behavior altogether but to learn how to control it. If you chose to read this book, perhaps you are ready to make a commitment to change.

The members of the Procrastinators Support Group wrote a pledge that they recite at the beginning of each meeting. It helps put them in the right frame of mind for making changes in their behavior. When you are ready to change directions and get off the road to procrastination, you might consider making this pledge to yourself.

*"I am a person who sometimes chooses to put things off for a while.*

*"I usually have a good reason, even if I am not fully aware of it.*

*"I have to admit that procrastination works for me some of the time, but I want to change.*

*"I can learn to do things differently."*

## Roadmap to Improvement

As you read through this book and practice the various exercises, you will learn a great deal about your tendency to procrastinate. Your improved self-awareness will put you in a stronger position to make changes that last. By the time you get to the last chapter, you will be ready to begin your program for reducing procrastination in the important areas of your life. When you get there, you will be prompted to state your reasons for changing your behavior. The examples provided throughout the book will give you some ideas of why other people choose to stop procrastinating. To initiate your plan for self-improvement you will need to pick a place to start. Once you have a better feel for the types of procrastination that plague you, it will be easier to pick a target to change. Along with choosing a target, you will be coached to set a realistic goal for improvement. This will keep you from trying to do too much too fast and risk getting overwhelmed. Finally, you will have a chance to plan how to take your first steps in the direction of change. As you read through these chapters, keep some notes on your reasons for change, goals, and ideas for how to get started.

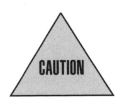

There is a good chance that you will stop reading this book even though you think it is a good idea to continue. You might tell yourself that you will read it later or after you have finished some other task. It is very possible that you will get busy and forget all about it. Or you might tell yourself that because your procrastination score was so high, there is no hope for change. Until you have learned a few skills for sticking with tasks, you will have to recognize and resist the urge to procrastinate.

In the next chapter you'll find a collection of Shortcuts to help you get started down a better path. They are temporary measures, just to help you make some quick progress. The remaining chapters have both Shortcuts and Changing Directions strategies for making bigger and more lasting changes. It has taken a while for you to become a procrastinator, so it will take a while to learn a different coping strategy. It is easier to start small by using the Shortcuts in situations that you can more easily master. Build your confidence and prove to yourself that you can make small changes. Once you have done that, you can work on making them more permanent.

If you have made it through this chapter, you are already heading down a better path. Keep going. Change is just around the corner.

# 2 | Shortcuts to Help You Get Started

**Directions:**

START: Know your tendency to procrastinate and outsmart it.

➡ Avoid getting seduced by procrastination.

➡ Get off the guilt trip.

➡ Learn how to stop making excuses.

END: Take your first positive step in the right direction.

## Your Journey Begins

Through the exercises in this book you will follow a new road map to your destination. You will gain a deeper understanding of why you procrastinate, and you will learn new strategies for preventing procrastination. You can overcome your personal roadblocks to taking action. All you have to do is stop being a passenger. Take the wheel. Handle your underlying problem and get back on the road to accomplishment. To get started on this new path you will have to learn a few things. First, you must recognize that you have a choice. You have control over the path you take—to procrastinate or not. Second, you must learn to recognize the urge to procrastinate so you can control it. Third, you have to figure out what drives you off the path to your goals. Fourth, to make progress you must acknowledge that procrastination works for you in the short run and that you will always be tempted to take that path to avoid tasks. You can change your ways if you commit to learning to do things differently.

## Let's Be Honest

You know you're a procrastinator. That's why you're reading this book. This chapter and the following ones are full of strategies for outsmarting procrastination. Your tendency to procrastinate, however, could keep you from using them to make needed changes. If you hesitate, put off, delay, resist, or avoid reading this book, you will miss out on a chance to put procrastination behind you. The first Shortcuts, therefore, provide some quick fixes for dealing with the urge to procrastinate on reading this book.

▶▶ Shortcuts for

### Resisting the Urge to Procrastinate on This Book

- Keep this book out in the open. If you can see it, you are more likely to read it.

- Don't set an unrealistic goal about reading it, such as that you will read it all this week or this month or you will read it before you do anything else.

- Plan to read only a page at a time.

- Keep it handy. Read it only during television commercials.

- Read it while you eat your lunch.

- Keep it in the bathroom and read it when you have time to spare.

- Don't tell yourself that you "have to" read it. Tell yourself that you want to read it.

Throughout this chapter are common problems encountered by most procrastinators and Shortcuts for maneuvering around them. Keep in mind that the Shortcuts are just that—quick ways to get around obstacles but not permanent solutions. You will have to read on in the book to learn new skills for overcoming the problems that underlie procrastination.

## "I'm Just Not Feeling It"

Waiting for the right mood? Procrastinators are kidding themselves when they believe they will recognize the right time to get moving. The assumption is that a feeling will come over you that will lift you off the couch, turn off the TV, and take procrastination off the table. The feeling is motivation. The problem is that motivation is often unpredictable and elusive. It is an emotion. It comes and goes, and you can't always count on its being around when you need it. It is true that when motivation is present procrastination is not an issue. But sometimes we have to take action even when motivation is low.

The right mood is not always needed to take action. You can do a chore when you are in a bad mood just as easily as when you are in a good mood. In fact, sometimes a bad mood can give you the energy you need to get things done. For example, if I'm angry with my husband in the evening and don't want to be in the same room with him, I will delay going to bed by cleaning the kitchen or doing the laundry. The anger energizes me to scrub and sweep with vigor. On the other hand, if I am in a particularly good mood, I don't want to do chores. I would rather play. You can't rely on mood as your guide for taking action.

▶▶ Shortcuts for
## Low Motivation

Sometimes when we are "not feeling it," we have to psych ourselves up by finding a reason to be motivated. Think of something you are procrastinating on right now and consider three reasons that it would be a good idea to stop delaying and get moving. Pick the reason that means the most to you. Repeat it to yourself as you prepare to take the first step. Write down your reasons and tell another person why it is important for you to stop procrastinating. When you do this, you are using your mind to guide you rather than your emotions. You're being smart. You know what to do.

The Procrastinators Support Group members have all used this Shortcut to give their motivation a boost. Here's what their lists of reasons looked like on a recent occasion. The reason in **bold** type is the one each picked as most important.

*Arthur is procrastinating on finishing a report for the support group.*

Reasons to stop procrastinating:

1. "So I don't have to think about it anymore."
2. "So people will not get mad at me for not doing it."
3. **"So I don't have to humiliate myself by showing up without it."**

*Olivia is putting off calling businesses to make donations for the church raffle.*

Reasons to get on the ball with this:

1. **"It's important to the church."**
2. "People are counting on me."
3. "I said I would do it."

*Bob is avoiding calls from his ex-wife's attorney.*

Reasons to take the calls:

1. "To get him off my back."
2. "To get my ex-wife off my back."
3. **"So my daughter doesn't think I'm a loser."**

*Freddie has not started on his term paper that is due next week.*

Reasons to get to work:

1. "I don't want to fail the class."
2. **"I hate getting stressed out at the last minute."**
3. "I promised myself a reward when I am done with it."

*Evelyn has avoided doing her laundry.*

Reasons to get it done:

1. **"I'm out of underwear."**
2. "The laundry room stinks."
3. "My mother is nagging me."

## ✑ A Personal Note

*I hate cleaning toilets. I have tried waiting for the right mood to clean the toilets in my house. It never comes. I have to clean the toilets because they need it even when I am not in the right mood. Come to think of it, what would be the right mood for toilet cleaning? When I think about it, I can't imagine what that feeling would be. Maybe fear can be a feeling that motivates me, such as the fear that a visitor will see or smell it and be grossed out. Maybe disgust is a feeling that would motivate me to clean them. When I think about being in the mood to clean toilets, it's not that I wait until I am fearful or disgusted enough to clean. I imagine a positive feeling coming over me that will make me want to drop everything I am doing, grab the toilet brush, and go for it. But I just don't see that happening. Sometimes I have to do things because they need to be done even when I am not in the mood. I guess, like death and taxes, the only certainty is that even if it's not dirty toilets, there will always be things to do we would rather avoid.*

# Don't Get Seduced

Procrastinating thoughts can be very seductive. They make promises they can't keep, such as "Just finish watching the movie. You can do the dishes later." They promise you plenty of time to catch up: "It won't take that long to read the materials. You have all afternoon to get it done." Procrastinating thoughts try to boost your ego: "You are so quick, you will have no trouble. Take it easy a little longer." They sugar-coat everything to make it seem easy: "You can run to the store later. There won't be any traffic, any lines, or any other obstacles to slow you down. In fact, you may not have to go to the store at all. You can make do with what you have."

Do any of these thoughts sound familiar? You are both the seducer and the seduced. Listen for that voice in your head. You can catch it trying to veer you off in the wrong direction. Just remember that if you can convince yourself to procrastinate, delay, or avoid, you can convince yourself to do the opposite.

## ▶▶ Shortcuts for
## Seductive Thoughts

Don't fall for it. Recognize the voice of seduction and don't let it manipulate you. You are smarter than that. You know when your inner procrastinator is lying to you, manipulating you, and making promises it can't keep. Practice these rational responses to your inner procrastinator:

- "I am procrastinating. That is what I do, but I want to change."

- "I may be able to wait a short while, but I can't keep putting things off."

- "I'm not going to accomplish what I need to do if I keep delaying."

- "Cut it out. Don't do what you always do."

- "Get moving. Take the right path."
- "If I can convince myself to stop, I can convince myself to go."

Evelyn's inner procrastinator is a seductive little thing. When she is engrossed in a television show and her thoughts start wandering to things she has to do, the voice of her inner procrastinator whispers, "Don't worry about it. It can wait." "You have time. It's not a big deal." If her mom comes into the room and tells her for the third time to turn off the TV and do the dishes, Evelyn sometimes slips and gives voice to her inner procrastinator: "Don't worry about it, Mom." That is usually all it takes to start an argument that Evelyn can't win. Evelyn has learned to suppress those words so that she avoids being scolded by her mom.

Evelyn has learned the hard way that waiting until the last minute at school can get her in trouble with her grades. Over the last few years of college, she has put off assignments so long that she forgot all about them. Getting a few Fs really made an impression on her. She knows from experience that letting herself get seduced with thoughts like "I'll worry about it later" is not a good strategy, so when she catches herself doing that, she makes an effort to put the assignment on the top of her homework pile. When she is back at home on break from school, she still gives in to her procrastination. Perhaps this is because she has not suffered any big consequences for it. Her mother nags and her siblings criticize her, but she has gotten used to that. She knows that she is procrastinating, but she hates to do chores and is not ready to change in that area.

Dorothea read a philosophy book once that emphasized living in the moment and getting the most out of life. When she finds herself getting stressed out by bills or by balancing her checkbook, she takes a deep breath, tells herself to live in the moment, breathe in the good, and breathe out the bad. This makes her feel better, so she puts away the bills and the checkbook for another day. While there is nothing wrong with living in the moment and trying to get the most out of life, Dorothea has used these ideas to justify procrastinating on things that cause tension. They are seductive because they convince her that she is just following the guidance of spiritual leaders. When she is honest with herself, she sees that she is using this not just to cope but also to avoid.

# Get Off the Guilt Trip

Most procrastinators get upset with themselves for procrastinating. Some beat themselves up with words like *loser* and *lazy*. Some burden themselves by viewing tasks as demands or obligations. They tell themselves that they "should" or "must" or "have to" get things done. Many procrastinators are very self-critical, but the harsh words do not motivate them to get busy. To take a step away from procrastination, you might try to recognize the guilt trips you take and try one of the Shortcuts in the next section to begin going in a new direction.

## Shoulds, Have Tos, and Musts

*Should* is one of those words that can take all the fun or interest or desire out of even the potentially most enjoyable tasks. It brings to mind thoughts of obligation, responsibility, duty, and requirement. Dyed-in-the-wool procrastinators, although usually responsible, innately feel the desire to pull away from an activity if it falls into one of those categories. If you are trying to motivate yourself by telling yourself what you "should" do, you may be making it worse.

Dorothea kept telling herself that she "should" paint her living room before her father saw it again. This would allow her to avoid embarrassment or criticism from him as well as his disappointment in her. When Dorothea asked herself what other reasons there might be to paint the living room, the answers were "because I think it is ugly the way it is, I like bolder colors in my living space, my furniture does not go well with the current color, and when I change something in my home it makes me feel better." These are all very good reasons to paint the living room. They motivate and excite her rather than fill her with dread. Try this yourself the next time you are procrastinating on something you think you "should" do.

▶▶ Shortcuts for
## Stopping the *Shoulds*

When you hear yourself say or think the word *should,* try to rephrase it. Think of a reason to take action other than because you "should" do so. Use those other reasons to motivate yourself into action. Here are a few examples of *should*s and their alternatives.

*"I should stop procrastinating."* "I will feel better about myself if I make some progress."

*"I should be on top of things."* "I like feeling organized."

*"People should honor their obligations."* "Doing what I promised to do makes me feel responsible and respectable."

*"I have to get an A."* "I want to do as well as I can on this test."

*"I must get this done today."* "I will start working on this today and try to finish it."

*"It has to be done right or not at all."* "I want to do my best on this."

## Self-Criticism

It is very common for procrastinators to get angry with themselves for stalling, avoiding, delaying, putting off, ignoring, and engaging in other forms of procrastination. They might call themselves names such as *lazy* or *worthless*. These are usually labels they heard from their parents or their teachers. The questions they ask themselves—such as "Why am I such a slob?" or "What's wrong with me?" or "Why am I so lazy?"—suggest they buy into these criticisms, Self-criticism is rarely motivating. Beating yourself up with words can lead to self-loathing, discouragement, low mood, and loss of confidence, none of which will increase your motivation to take action.

Another form of negative self-talk is defeatist thinking. When you start to believe "That's just how I am. I'm never going to change. I can't help it," you are accepting the status quo.

Recognizing the self-defeating nature of self-criticism, the members of Chapter 121 of the Procrastinators Support Group made a master list of all of the self-critical statements made during the meetings. When new members of the group told their story and criticized themselves, the ledger they kept would be opened and shown to the new member. The new member would be asked to write down his or her self-critical statement. This was their way of letting the new person know that he or she was not alone in thinking such thoughts.

Their ledger included statements such as those listed in the following box. Read through the list and mark the ones that sound familiar or add your own.

---

### Procrastinators Support Group Chapter 121
### Ledger of Self-Critical Thoughts

- "I'm a lazy bum."

- "I'm worthless."

- "I have no purpose."

- "I'll never change."

- "I hate myself when I procrastinate."

- "I don't have what it takes."

- "I'm a useless human being."

- "I can't help it. I was just born lazy."

- "My mom was right. I'll never amount to anything."

- "There is no excuse for my behavior."

You should read Chapter 5, on self-doubt, and Chapter 3, on avoidance as a way of coping, to learn more about how to control negative self-talk. The Shortcut that follows is a tool for getting you to slow down and briefly think through your tendency to be self-critical. The hope is that if you consider the questions listed you might be able to dismiss negative thoughts that are making you procrastinate.

▶▶ Shortcuts for
## Self-Criticism

To help you control your self-criticism about procrastination, try asking yourself these questions:

1. "What good does it do for me to criticize myself?"

2. "How does it help me?"

3. "Does it make me feel more motivated?"

4. "Does it inspire me?"

5. "Does it put me in a good mood?"

If self-criticism doesn't help you, it's time to get off that familiar road and try a new path. If you were capable of opening this book, you are capable of more. If you read this far, you can go a little further. If you don't like being a procrastinator, then you have found a good reason to change.

### Procrastination with an Extra Layer of Guilt

Not all procrastinators feel guilty when they procrastinate. The ones who do feel guilty about it find that their procrastination becomes unpleasant and difficult to enjoy. Arthur finds this confusing. On the one hand he knows he is choosing to procrastinate instead of working. On the other hand, he feels guilty about it. The guilt does not motivate him. It makes him feel worse, but it doesn't make him stop procrastinating. Arthur's strategy is to distract himself from the guilt by finding something fun to do. Once he gets engrossed in a television show or is out doing things with his family or friends, he forgets about the guilt until something reminds him of what needs to be done. Once reminded, he tells himself, "I'll take care of it tomorrow," even though he knows that there is only about a 25% chance that he will actually do it.

Making you feel guilty about your procrastination is a strategy often used with children by teachers, parents, coaches, and clergy. When you grow up, the guilt trip becomes part of your inner thoughts when you procrastinate. While you resisted doing chores or homework when you were a kid, you still took in the words of the important people in your life that made you feel guilty about procrastinating. Those words stuck in your mind and eventually became your own words, so when you procrastinate as an adult, the guilt-inducing lecture pops back into your mind. It gets reinforced if you share your adult life with people who try to make you feel guilty when they think you are procrastinating. The more susceptible to guilt you are, the less you can enjoy a relaxing moment of laziness. It can make procrastination almost not worth it.

## ⚲ A Personal Note

*If guilt inducement worked, then procrastination would never be a problem for people who came from cultures or religions where guilt was used to motivate. I'm Catholic. Guilt for not taking action has been just as much a theme in my life as guilt for doing something bad. I can't walk by litter on the street without feeling bad for not picking it up right away. When I work with a group on a project, I can't not do my part. I can't say no when I know I have the time and ability to help out others even when I would rather relax.*

*Raising three sons has made it worse. When I was a den mother for my youngest son's Cub Scout troop, I had to demonstrate responsibility if I was going to teach it. As coach of my middle son's soccer team, I had to model the value of working hard, doing your part for your team, and not slacking off. As the "water mom" for my oldest son's high school band, I made myself leave work early on many Friday afternoons to fill water coolers with water and ice when I would rather have gone for a massage or a movie or taken a nap before the boys came home from school. As a mom who tried to teach my sons to balance work and play, I had to model a good work ethic. They were naturally very good at playing. Add this to my personal rule that I have to practice what I preach, and the result is guilt when I don't toe the line. I think this is what keeps me from enjoying a lazy afternoon. It doesn't keep me from procrastinating. It just keeps me from enjoying it. Many of my Catholic friends say the same thing. They feel bad, but it doesn't stop their procrastination.*

Negative emotions like guilt and negative thinking like self-criticism can affect your actions. They keep procrastination going instead of stopping it. You will learn more about how this works in the next chapter. For now, suffice it to say that because it only makes you feel bad and doesn't solve procrastination, you are just spinning your wheels when you follow procrastination with a healthy serving of guilt. You can increase your chances of overcoming your tendency to procrastinate if you can get past the habit of beating yourself up. Many more productive strategies are described in the chapters that follow. Read ahead and pick one that works for you. Stop the guilt trip and find a more productive path.

## Stop Making Excuses

Some procrastinators have dysfunctional beliefs about when it is time to stop procrastinating and start taking action. These beliefs help justify their procrastination. They are called *dysfunctional* because they make procrastination worse, not better. Some examples of dysfunctional beliefs about procrastination are in the following box.

## Dysfunctional Beliefs about Procrastination

- "I need to be in the right mood."
- "It's not the right time."
- "I'll know when it is time to do it."
- "I need to think about it some more."
- "I'm just not feeling it."
- "I'm not in the right place."
- "I'll get to it when I get to it."

Do any of these ideas sound familiar to you? They are quite common among procrastinators. Now let's look a little more closely at the beliefs that tell us we should procrastinate to reveal why they are not to be trusted. Besides the fact that they tend to prolong procrastination rather than end it, there are a number of problems with these types of beliefs. First of all, these beliefs are dysfunctional because they are not usually based on facts. They are based more on feelings. There is no perfect time to get started on a project like filing your taxes, writing a term paper, or cleaning your kitchen. You don't have to feel ready to get started. Your mind and body work even when the timing is not ideal. There is no brain mechanism that signals when the time is right to stop procrastinating. Dorothea has been waiting for the right time to paint her living room for nearly a year. She has not been in the mood or has not felt right about the color. She thinks that the urge to paint will be there one morning and when it does she will take care of it. This strategy hasn't worked for her so far.

Another problem with these thoughts that make us procrastinate is that they suggest we have no control over when to take action. They imply that we have to wait patiently until the feeling comes or the time is right. We can't force it. We can't schedule projects ahead of time, planning to tackle them when it is most convenient for us. We have to wait around until our unconscious mind sends a signal to our conscious awareness, which translates into a feeling that motivates us to get off our butts and take care of business. This is nonsense. We *do* have control over when to take action. We can choose to get going or not. Instead of waiting on some unpredictable force to make up its mind, we can take control and take action!

Dorothea doesn't have to wait for the right moment or the right feeling. She can decide that next Saturday at 9:00 A.M. she will go to the paint store and buy the supplies she needs. She can decide that Sunday morning she will get up early and start preparing the walls for paint. She does not have to wait for the magic feeling. She is smart and able and can make decisions on her own. She just doesn't know this yet.

## ▶▶ Shortcuts for
## Ending the Excuses

1. Recognize what you are doing. Admit to yourself that you are making excuses.

2. Take control of the situation by making the decision to take action.

3. Whatever the task is, tell yourself that it has to be done. Waiting another day will not make the task easier to do.

4. Make an effort even if it is a small one.

5. Pat yourself on the back for getting that far.

Dorothea's dad called and asked how her home repairs were coming along. She lied about it and told him things were going well. She hates lying to her dad, but she was embarrassed to say that the walls of her apartment were still an ugly shade of purplish gray. They talked about him coming to visit her for her birthday. This created a feeling of panic because her birthday was only a month away and there was little chance that Dorothea could get her apartment done in time. She didn't discourage his visit, but she didn't encourage it either.

When Dorothea got off the phone, she knew she had to stop making excuses. She was running out of time. She looked around the apartment at her ugly walls that did not match her furniture. She told herself it was time to get with it. She made a commitment to pick out a color for the wall over the next week. If she was still uncertain by next week, she would just paint the walls white—not her favorite color, but it would work. Dorothea felt better that she had made a plan for taking a first step. She promised herself a peppermint mocha latte at the coffee bar around the corner after she made a decision on the paint color.

Now that you have taken a few Shortcuts to get you off the path of procrastination, it is time to work on the problems that underlie your procrastination. The next chapter is about avoidance and the reasons that people use this way to cope. You will hear about several of the support group members' tendency to avoid stressful tasks or situations as their way of dealing with discomfort. These people have learned to move in a different direction. Use their strategies for confronting discomfort. They could help you on your journey away from procrastination.

# 3 | What Are You Afraid Of?

**Directions:**

> **START:** Figure out whether fear is making you procrastinate.
>
> ⟶ Learn how fear leads to procrastination.
>
> ⟶ Find out whether fear of the unknown is holding you back.
>
> ⟶ Reduce catastrophizing.
>
> **END:** Learn how to stop scaring yourself.

*"I'm afraid it's going to be … unpleasant, uncomfortable, embarrassing, painful."*

*"I'm scared to find out … bad news, that I didn't succeed, that others are disappointed in me."*

*"I don't want to talk to her because … she might be mad, I might hurt her feelings, it will be awkward."*

*"What if I make a change and … I fail, it doesn't work out, it turned out to be a bad idea?"*

*"I don't know … what will happen, if it's the right thing to do, how it will turn out?"*

Fear is a powerful emotion and one of the most common reasons that people procrastinate. We begin our discussion of the various forces behind procrastination and the subtypes of procrastinators by talking first about fear and about how procrastination helps us avoid fearful, scary, or stressful situations.

Fear can take many different forms. Emotionally, fear can feel like anxiety, stress, mistrust, worry, discomfort, nervousness, concern, apprehension, and even paranoia. Physically, fear can show itself as muscle tension, headaches, stomachaches, chest pain, heart palpitations, excessive sweating, dizziness, nausea, skin rashes, trembling, shaking, ringing in the ears, and many other uncomfortable sensations. Fear is fueling our thoughts when we imagine the worst-case scenario; when we think, "What if ...?" and imagine a bad outcome; when we are concerned about what others will think of us; when we anticipate humiliation or embarrassment; and when we fear the unknown. Fear also shows in our actions. It makes us avoid difficult people and stressful situations. And it makes us procrastinate when the outcome is uncertain, dreaded, scary, or likely to be unpleasant. Kendall is afraid of hurting Lance's feelings, so she puts off telling him she isn't interested. Evelyn is afraid she will be in trouble, so she doesn't tell her superior at the library that she broke the copier. Dorothea fears her father's disapproval, so she puts off painting her living room because she thinks she might not be able to do it perfectly. Freddie thinks the news will be bad, so he doesn't return his mother's phone call. Does fear make you procrastinate? Look over Changing Directions 3 to see if it describes you.

---

↻ Changing Directions 3
## Is Fear Your Problem?

Fear may be one of your reasons for procrastination if

- Thinking about the task makes you feel uncomfortable.
- You worry a lot about how it will turn out.
- You hesitate to get started for fear you'll mess it up.
- You wonder if you can handle it.
- When you try to do it you feel tense, your heart races, or you start to feel hot.
- You think people will criticize, reject, or laugh at you.

Fear *is not* your problem if you procrastinate because

- You are feeling lazy.
- You are tired.
- You are feeling discouraged.
- You just can't concentrate.
- You would rather do something more fun.


## Thoughts, Feelings, and Actions

Procrastination is an action. What inspires you to procrastinate is the combination of two things. One is your belief that taking action now will be unpleasant in some way. The second is your emotions, the feelings that get stirred up inside when you think of taking action on something you would rather not do.

**Your negative thoughts + Your emotional reaction**
↓
**Procrastination**

Here are some examples of how common thoughts and the feelings that accompany them can lead you to procrastinate.

*"I don't know what to do"* + Anxiety
↓
Procrastination

*"I can't deal with this right now"* + Fatigue
↓
Procrastination

*"I hate having to do things like this"* + Irritation
↓
Procrastination

> *"This is going to be so messed up"* + Dread
> ↓
> Procrastination

If you can identify the thought and the feeling that together are leading you to procrastinate, you can choose another way to cope. For example, if you recognize that the real problem is you are not sure what to do first, you can cope by asking someone else for his or her opinion, by reading instructions, or by making a list of your options.

If you are too exhausted to take on a difficult task, rest for a while and then go back to it. If you are irritated because you are being forced to do something unpleasant that you would rather avoid, find a way to make the task less unpleasant, like getting someone fun to do it with you. If you are procrastinating because you anticipate that the activity is going to be unpleasant or the outcome is going to be bad, take time to think about how you can make it turn out better. If there is no way to prevent it from being uncomfortable or negative, find a way to cope by thinking of ways you have coped with unpleasantness in the past.

Could this work for you? Keep reading and you will learn many different ways to cope when your negative thoughts and emotions are making you avoid something you would rather not do.

## How Fear Can Get the Best of You

Emotion has a way of coloring our views of our world, our futures, and ourselves. This is what cognitive therapists like Dr. Aaron Beck, the developer of cognitive therapy, call the *cognitive triad*—three important areas of our lives. When we are afraid, the world looks scary. When we are apprehensive, our future seems questionable. When we are anxious, we doubt our ability to cope. When these feelings and thoughts are strong enough, they can lead to procrastination. While we are procrastinating we have more time to think. The more we think, the worse the situation can seem. That raises anxiety and strengthens procrastination as a way of coping.

Actions—
procrastinate, avoid

Thoughts—
"I don't know how to
do it. I'm going to mess
it up."

Feelings—
tense, anxious, fearful

It is a vicious cycle, but it is a cycle that can be broken. In general, you can break the cycle by changing the way you view a situation so that you are no longer scaring yourself. You can also learn to lower the intensity of your fear, dread, nervousness, or apprehension so that these emotions stop fueling your negative thoughts. (There are exercises throughout the book to help you do this.) You can also learn to change your actions and stop procrastinating even when you feel anxious about taking action. Chapter 2 covered a variety of ways that you can begin to change your actions. In each of the remaining chapters there will be lots of suggestions for addressing your thoughts, feelings, and actions. When you change any one of these components, the others will change on their own.

Actions—
Take action, make some
progress, give it a try

Thoughts—
"Get started. It doesn't
have to be perfect."

Feelings—concern, encouraged

For example, Freddie called his mom to ask about her MRI results even though he was scared and was relieved to know that she was OK. When Arthur stopped assuming the group was going to find fault with his report, he calmed down and finished it. Evelyn took a deep breath, calmed herself, and then walked into her supervisor's office to tell him it was her fault the copier was broken. She was glad she had gotten it off her chest. Freddie changed his actions, Arthur changed his thoughts, and Evelyn changed her feelings. In each case, the cycle of procrastination was broken.

This chapter will focus more on changing your thought processes than on changing your behavior. You will learn how to recognize and straighten out your thinking when you are "freaking yourself out" about taking action. This will be done by systematically analyzing your thoughts and identifying distortions. If you can pick out your distorted thoughts, you can change them by making them more accurate and less emotional. This will become clearer as you read on.

## Don't Let Fear of the Unknown Hold You Back

The hesitation, delay, and avoidance that are typical of procrastination are often fueled by a fear of the unknown. When you wait to take action because you are not sure how things will turn out, it is the unknown that is holding you back. You may not be certain what to expect, but you imagine that it could be something unpleasant, stressful, uncomfortable, or difficult.

Bob had been reluctant to join the Procrastinators Support Group even though he knew he was in great need of help. He had heard that self-help groups are full of people who whine and complain and that they put you on the spot and make you cry. "Until Arthur told me how these meetings worked, I wasn't sure it was for me. I figured they all held hands and sang 'Kumbaya.'" Not knowing how the group was run kept Bob from joining for a long time.

Polly needed to lose some weight. She heard that there was a counselor at the YMCA in her neighborhood who could evaluate her body size and put her on a personalized exercise program. She wasn't sure how they did it, but she had seen a TV special about measuring body fat, and she didn't want anyone pinching her belly fat or dunking her in a tank of water just to tell her that she had a lot of fat. She knew she was fat. Not knowing how the program works is still keeping Polly away from the YMCA.

Sally thought about taking a night class to learn how to speak Spanish. She kept putting it off because she didn't know what they made you do in class, but she definitely didn't want to have to stand up in front of everyone and embarrass herself. She thought about getting audiotapes or CDs that taught you how to make conversation in Spanish, but they were much more expensive than the night class. The class is offered every semester. At the beginning of every term she promises to sign up next time. This has been her pattern for several years.

People procrastinate even on activities that are really good ideas when they are not sure how things will turn out. Sometimes they put off small things like getting a new hairstyle because they are not certain how it will look. Or they delay getting a pet because they think it could be too much work. Sometimes the procrastination is over really big changes, like deciding whether to get married. A person who is uncertain about how something will turn out will put it off until he has had more time to think about it. Taking time to think things through is generally a good plan, but it works only if you eventually make a decision about how you want to proceed and then follow through with that decision. Most of the time we don't do this when we procrastinate. Instead we put the idea aside with the intention of getting back to it another day. True procrastinators will recognize this for what it is, another delay tactic.

## Fortune–Telling

The thought process that makes you procrastinate when you are afraid of the unknown is called *fortune-telling*. Although you are uncertain what the outcome will be, you "get a feeling" that it may not turn out the way you want. Fear of the unknown can be mistaken for instinct. People will say they have a bad feeling about something, so they avoid it. They tell themselves that it "doesn't feel right," so they put it off until it feels better. In the previous examples, Polly doesn't really know if going to the gym at the YMCA will be a humiliating experience, but just in case it might be, she keeps putting it off. She has a bad feeling about it, but it is more than instinct. She is actually imagining a situation where she will feel embarrassed by the counselor measuring her fat. It is not that she thinks they will announce her body measurements on the loudspeaker or tell the other women in the gym. She knows they are probably very professional about it, but since she isn't exactly sure how they measure fat, she has a feeling it will be humiliating for another person to know how much she weighs or to know just how much bigger her thighs are than everyone else's at the gym. She anticipates feeling bad, so she procrastinates in going even though she really wants to start exercising. She tells herself that after she loses 15 pounds and starts walking on her own, she will go to the gym. That way the counselor will be impressed that she has made progress, she will have better stamina in walking, and her thighs will be less embarrassing. While this sounds like a great plan, Polly never seems to be able to get started on it.

When Polly imagines embarrassment over going to the counselor at the YMCA, she is making a fortune-telling error. It is an error in logic, because Polly has no idea how the measurements are made or how confidential they might be because she has made no effort to find out how it works. Instead of continuing to use fortune-telling to guide your decisions about when to act, try Changing Directions 4. It will show you how to deal with fortune-telling.

---

↺ Changing Directions 4
## Dealing with Fortune-Telling

**Focus:** *Fear of the unknown*—Procrastinating because you are not sure how things will turn out, but you assume they might turn out badly.

**Thinking Error:** *Fortune-telling*—Letting your uncertainty lead you to assume there could be a bad outcome.

**Goal:** Stop relying on gut-level feelings or instincts to guide your choices. Get information, collect data, or gather facts and then decide what to do.

> *Solution 1.* **Read the other palm,** check out another crystal ball, shake up the eight ball, and look again at the prediction or make another guess. Fortune-telling usually stops at the first scary idea that comes to mind. Let your mind wander more and consider other possible outcomes. Perhaps there are others that are less frightening. Once you have had a chance to consider the options, decide which is most likely to occur. Just because your scary thought seemed believable at first does not mean it is the most likely outcome.
>
> *Solution 2.* **Get information.** If the future is unknown, ask others, read about it, surf the Internet for answers, or observe how others do it before you take action.

In Polly's case, other possible outcomes are that the counselor will evaluate her in a private room and keep the information confidential, Polly will be able to choose which method of measurement is used, the counselor will be sensitive to Polly's embarrassment and make her feel better, or, if others overhear her measurements, they will offer encouragement since they are all in the program to lose weight. It is also possible that if someone with poor manners makes fun of her, Polly will be able to handle the situation and not let it keep her from her goals. When Polly thought about it, she thought the most likely outcome was that the counselor would handle her body measurements in a professional manner. She decided to get more information by going to the YMCA and talking with the fitness counselor before signing up for the program. Once she heard an explanation of their program, she was less concerned about embarrassment. She saw the women exercising in a group. They were just as fat as she was, so she felt right at home.

### ꙭ *A Personal Note*

*There is a big difference between knowing how to change and actually doing it. If knowing how to change automatically led to improvement, then mental health professionals would all be perfect people. Trust me; we're not perfect. For example, I know all the rules for losing weight. I know what to eat and not eat. I know how important it is to exercise. I know how many calories I would have to not eat or to burn to lose a pound. You would think that all that knowledge would keep me away from desserts or would get me to the gym more regularly. It doesn't. All that knowledge helps me make good choices most of the time. It doesn't make me give up desserts, but it does keep me from overdoing it. It makes me not order fries with my cheeseburger and skip the mayonnaise on my sandwiches. Knowledge also helps me keep healthy habits like eating fruits and vegetables and drinking plenty of water. My point is that gaining knowledge is a good start and will help you develop good habits, but knowledge alone is not enough for complete and total change. We are human, and so we are less than perfect. We have urges and emotions that affect our thoughts and actions like my urge for chocolate when I'm feeling stressed.*

*If you are like me, you will be able to use the information in this book to begin to change. It will start with becoming more self-aware. With self-awareness comes choice. You will be able to choose to use your usual ways of coping, such as procrastination, or choose to use one of the skills from this book. Try to put the skills you learn into action as often as you can. Know that the urges or emotions or instincts that make you procrastinate will not go away all at once. Make your plan be to try to procrastinate less today than you did yesterday and to try to procrastinate less tomorrow than you do today.*

## Mind Reading

Donna hasn't spoken to her grandmother in more than a year. She has avoided her grandmother's calls because she knows her grandmother would be opposed to her divorce, which was just finalized. Donna's mother has urged Donna to talk to her grandmother before the family gets together for Thanksgiving. Donna doesn't think she could bear her grandmother's disapproval. That is why she keeps procrastinating on calling her. Her mother tells her that it will not be that bad and that the grandmother understands Donna's reasons for getting out of the marriage, but that does not comfort Donna.

Donna hates confrontation with someone she loves. She will argue with bill collectors, demand service in a store when she is being ignored, and even get aggressive with others to defend her friends or family members. In these situations she doesn't care what those people think of her. When it comes to family or friends, Donna clams up. She doesn't want the important people in her life to hate her or be angry with her. She thinks it would be awful if her loved ones thought badly of her, so she goes out of her way to avoid making a bad impression. That means that sometimes she has to keep her opinions to herself, avoid discussion of unpleasant topics, hide her true feelings, and go along with things against her better judgment.

Donna is not worried that her family members or friends will yell at her or criticize her openly. She can handle direct attacks. She worries that people will hold negative opinions of her, feel disappointed in her, or disapprove of her actions without telling her. That is why she has avoided talking with her grandmother. She loves her grandmother and respects her opinion. She believes her grandmother would be disappointed that Donna could not make her marriage work. She knows her grandmother is too kind to say so, but Donna thinks she will be able to hear the disappointment in her voice or see it in her eyes.

Making assumptions about what other people are thinking or feeling is called *mind reading*. It is another type of thinking error. If you are a mind reader, try some of the suggestions in Changing Directions 5.

---

↺ Changing Directions 5
## Getting Beyond Mind Reading

**Focus:** *Fear of the reactions of others*—Assuming that others will react in a negative way and avoiding such interactions.

**Thinking Error:** *Mind reading*—Making guesses about how other people feel and what they think about you even when they have not directly communicated their thoughts or feelings.

**Goal:** Recognize that you are not a mind reader. Use facts and not guesses to guide your actions. If you don't have enough information, ask questions before you jump to conclusions.

*Solution 1.* **Ask questions** instead of making assumptions that others are thinking badly of you. For example, if you lost your job, rather than assume that others think you are a pathetic loser, ask, "Are you disappointed in me?" "Do you think it's my fault?" "Are you mad at me?" Give them a chance to voice their opinions rather than assuming the worst.

*Solution 2.* **Test out your guesses** by voicing your concern. For example, if you have to tell your parents that you have decided to quit school, you might start the conversation talking about your fears, such as "I'm worried that you will be mad at me if I tell you what I want to do" or "I'm afraid to talk to you because I don't want you to be upset with me" or "I don't want you to be disappointed in me, but there is something I want to tell you."

*Solution 3.* **Stay off the defensive.** It is easy to feel defensive when you think someone is thinking badly of you. If you begin your conversation on the defensive, it will show in your tone of voice, your body language, and your choice of words. You might cause a conflict or a disagreement by coming off as harsh or argumentative. Try to keep your tone neutral or positive. Try not to defend yourself before there is an attack. For example, if you know you forgot to pay the phone bill and you imagine your partner will be angry with you, do not start the conversation off with "I know you're angry, but it's not my fault. I have a lot to do, and you should help more, and besides, you are the one that uses the phone more than me. Why can't you take care of it?" The best defense is not always a good offense.

*Solution 4*. **Consider the possibility that you are wrong.** Mind reading is the same as making assumptions. An assumption is just a guess, but many people jump to the conclusion that their guesses are accurate. When people are upset, they are usually poor guessers. So if you think your boss is going to fire you, rather than quit your job before she has a chance, consider the possibility that you might be wrong. Think it through before you react. The same would be true if you thought your boyfriend was not returning your call because he was seeing someone else. Don't freak out. Consider the possibility that you are being paranoid or insecure about the relationship before you confront him.

*Solution 5*. **Find a way to cope.** You might be putting off an important conversation because you anticipate a bad outcome, and maybe you are right. Turn your focus to how you would like to handle it if your prediction turns out to be correct. Make a plan for coping with a possible negative outcome. Donna, for example, feels pretty strongly that her grandmother is going to react badly, so she is turning her focus to how she will deal with the bad feelings that will probably linger.

It is normal for people to occasionally disapprove of one another, but both usually get over it with time. Think of the times when you have been disappointed in the actions of others but eventually let it go. Even if others react negatively to you, you can handle the situation and recover. Donna's grandmother might not like the fact that Donna is divorced, but she is unlikely to reject her forever. Donna can hear her grandmother's view, acknowledge her feelings, accept the disapproval, and try to get past it by mending the hurt feelings that linger. Donna is trying to use Solution 5 by coming up with a strategy for coping after her grandmother gives her that disappointed look. Remember that procrastination in talking with others just to avoid temporary discomfort is a short-term solution that can grow into a bigger problem if the avoidance goes on too long.

⏭ Shortcuts for
## Getting Past Hurt Feelings

Most hurt feelings will dissipate over time. However, you can keep those feelings fresh by thinking a lot about your hurts, retelling the hurtful story over and over to anyone who will listen, or thinking of ways to get revenge. An alternative strategy is to think of what you need so you can let go of the hurt feelings. Take charge of the hurt and find a way to soothe yourself. Find a short-term solution that will make you feel a little better today. It is always easier to add a positive than to take away a negative. Add a positive experience. Talk to a positive person. Do something kind for yourself or go out of your way to be nice to another person. Have some fun. You will find that the hurt will begin to lessen on its own.

# Stop Catastrophizing

Freddie anticipates disaster and tries to avoid it at all costs. He has a knack for imagining the worst-case scenario and accepting it as if it were a prophecy. The kinds of things that stir up Freddie's anxiety are hard classes, having to talk to people about stressful topics, and upcoming events with people that make him uncomfortable. Freddie would be the first to admit that what scares him most is not knowing what is going to happen next. He can deal with problems if he knows what to expect and has time to come up with a plan. He hates it when change is coming and he is not certain it will be a good thing. Freddie's mom is in poor health, and he is worried about her. His sister Agnes takes her to the doctor and tells him what the doctor said. The hardest part of this is waiting on test results. While he waits, he imagines the worst. So far, he has been wrong, and nothing seems to be seriously wrong with his mother other than her blood pressure being too high. Knowing this does not make Freddie worry any less. He is glad that Agnes takes care of his mother. He doesn't think he could handle it.

When you don't know what is going to happen next, it is easy to imagine the worst-case scenario. You fill in the blanks with fears, what ifs, and potential disasters. Your emotions make you jump to conclusions, and usually those conclusions are negative ones. The more you think about it, the more elaborate the disaster can become. This is called *catastrophizing*. Most catastrophizers do it with regularity, so it is easy to recognize. Freddie, for example, has always had a knack for imagining the worst. If you're inclined to catastrophize, try Changing Directions 6.

---

## ↺ Changing Directions 6
## Decatastrophizing Scary Thoughts

**Focus:** *Fear of what the future will bring*—Hoping for the best but preparing for the worst.

**Thinking Error:** *Catastrophizing*—Imagining the worst-case scenario and convincing yourself that it is likely to occur.

**Goal:** Stop scaring yourself by imagining catastrophes. Consider all possible outcomes and prepare for the most likely outcome.

*Solution 1.* Get perspective. How likely is it that the worst outcome will occur? Consider your experience. How often have you imagined the worst-case scenario and it never happened? Try to remember whether procrastinating made the situation turn out any better.

*Solution 2.* Consider the possibility that you are using catastrophic thinking as an excuse to continue procrastinating. When you are completely honest with yourself, does it become more obvious that a catastrophe is not very likely?

*Solution 3.* Try to gain perspective on the problem by asking yourself what advice you would give to a friend or family

---

member with the same fear. It is easier to give advice to others than to yourself. Talk to yourself in the mirror, write down your ideas, or use your imagination to address the scary thoughts. If you had to be strong for someone else who was scared, what advice would you give? Consider the options and pick the advice that applies to you. Listen to your own wisdom!

The next chapter covers difficulties with getting organized. Disorganization can make you think you have more time than you have to get things done. Disorganized procrastinators also think that tasks will take less time than turns out to be true. If this sounds like you, you probably find that you run out of time and can't get to or finish tasks. Maybe it's time to change strategies.

You are making good progress in your reading. Keep going. You should be pleased with yourself that you are taking steps toward overcoming your procrastination. Progress will come in small steps as you start to implement the strategies described in this book. The fact that you have made it to the end of Chapter 3 shows that you are already changing the way you deal with procrastination. You obviously have an open mind and are willing to learn how to change. These are big steps for most people. Congratulations! Keep up the good work!

# 4 ⎹ Are You Disorganized?

**Directions:**

| | |
|---|---|
| **START:** | Stop fooling yourself. |
| ➡ | Learn how to prioritize. |
| ➡ | Manage your time with realistic estimates. |
| ➡ | Avoid distractions. |
| **END:** | Take a step toward accomplishing weekly goals. |

A common practical problem that trips up procrastinators is disorganization. This chapter provides some practical solutions for common organization problems such as overestimating how much time you have for procrastination and underestimating how long it takes to get things done. Even if you think you are an organized person, read through at least the first section on how to stop fooling yourself. It might be the missing piece in your organizational strategy.

## Stop Fooling Yourself

Procrastinators often have an active fantasy life. The fantasies include how easy tasks will be and how much time there is to accomplish them. Fantasizing is how we convince ourselves that it is OK to procrastinate a little bit longer. Changing Directions 7 includes a list of common fantasies about procrastination. Find out how much you may be fooling yourself.

---

↻ Changing Directions 7

## The Fantasies behind Procrastination

Put a check next to the fantasies that run through your mind when you are faced with a task and have the urge to procrastinate.

- ❏ I can get it done.
- ❏ I work better under pressure.
- ❏ I have plenty of time.
- ❏ It won't take that long.
- ❏ Don't worry about it. It will get done.
- ❏ It's not a big deal.
- ❏ Someone else will do it.
- ❏ Someone else will help me.
- ❏ I always get it done eventually.
- ❏ So what if it doesn't get done?

*Count the number of items you checked.*

1 to 2 items: Suggests good self-confidence.

3 to 4 items: You may be fooling yourself a little. Be cautious.

5 to 6 items: Your overly positive self-talk is making you procrastinate.

7 to 10 items: You are definitely fooling yourself with these statements. It is time to develop a more realistic view.

---

Self-talk is very persuasive. If we tell ourselves often enough that we have all the time in the world, we will come to believe it. Even when time is running out, we can delude ourselves into thinking everything will be fine. In the last chapter you learned how negative thoughts and feelings could lead to procrastination. Positive thoughts, like those listed in Changing Directions 7, can work the same way.

You might be wondering what to think if both overly negative and unrealistically positive thoughts can cause procrastination. What else is there? The trick is to have realistic thoughts, those without distortion and without an overwhelming amount of emotion. You need to know exactly how much time you have to complete a job and make a realistic estimate of how much time it will take to finish it. You also need to be aware of all the other circumstances that can get in the way. With that information, you have a better chance of planning for how long you can afford to procrastinate and when you need to get back on task. Changing Directions 8 will give you some ideas for controlling unrealistic self-talk.

---

↺ Changing Directions 8
## Realistic Self-Talk

- **Hear it.** Learn to recognize unrealistic self-talk like the statements listed in Changing Directions 7. Write your most commonly used unrealistic statements on a note card and tape it to your mirror or desk or the dashboard of your car. If you see reminders like this, you will be more likely to catch these thoughts as they come to mind.
- **Know it.** Pay attention to how often your unrealistic self-talk is just an excuse to procrastinate. When you hear those statements in your mind, acknowledge that you are trying to justify or rationalize your procrastination. For example, when you think to yourself, "I have plenty of time," remember that this is what you always say when you want to procrastinate. Even if it is true that you have time, this is also the secret password that opens the door to stalling and avoiding.

---

- **Dismiss it.** See those thoughts for what they are. Don't let them fool you. You know that they are lies or excuses and you do not have to fall for them. If you know you are justifying your procrastination, turn it around and justify taking action.
- **Get real.** Admit that you are procrastinating. Decide when you will stop. Substitute more realistic statements for your fantasies, such as "I can get it done if I allow myself enough time" or "I don't think it will take that long, but I need to give that more thought."

"I can get that done in two minutes. It's not a big deal," Arthur said about reformatting the annual budget report. He always says, "It's not a big deal," and two minutes is his usual estimate. He's so convincing when he says it that the other support group members take him seriously. In reality, it always takes Arthur a lot more than 2 minutes to complete any computer or financial task, and it is almost always a big deal. He doesn't get asked to do the small stuff.

Bob heard Arthur's two-minute estimate and called him on it. "Arthur, you always say that, and it's rarely true."

"What do you mean?" asked Arthur.

"That whole 'I can get it done in two minutes' thing," answered Bob.

"Well, I guess you got me there. It will take more than two minutes. It takes me at least two minutes just to boot up my computer. Then I have to find my materials and figure out what I need to do; that's at least another 10 minutes. If my computer cooperates, I can probably make the changes in 20 minutes. If it doesn't cooperate, then it may be more like 45 minutes," admitted Arthur.

"Do you have 20 to 45 minutes to spare for this?" asked Dorothea. "Because it's really not that bad the way it is. I mean if it really took two minutes, I can see you making this change, but if we are talking about 45 minutes, it's not worth that much of your time."

Arthur thought about it. He didn't like to let people down,

especially after he so quickly spoke up about doing the reformat-ting. "On the other hand," he thought, "Bob was right. I always underestimate how long things will take, and I always overestimate how much time I have. It's tax season, and I don't even have enough time to stop for lunch at work. It doesn't make sense for me to agree to do a task that is not really necessary."

"Bob and Dorothea, thank you for stopping me," said Arthur. "You are both right. I do this all the time. I am my own worst enemy when it comes to time management. I don't have time to reformat that report, and I don't think we need it to file our tax report. You guys can help me break this habit by stopping me when I say I can do something in two minutes. It is a bad habit because when I say it I actually believe it myself even though it is not at all true. When I say the 'two-minute' thing and the 'it's no big deal' thing, I am just fooling myself. I really need to stop doing that."

The group applauded Arthur for his progress. They didn't mind that he could not reformat the report. They saw that he was struggling to stop his procrastination and that deciding not to do this task was a sign of progress.

Olivia runs into problems every Christmas season. She always makes great plans for buying and mailing gifts, baking and ship-ping cookies to her relatives, having people over to her home for a party, sending out cards, volunteering at the homeless shelter, and cooking an unforgettable Christmas dinner. She starts thinking about all that she wants to do when she sees the holiday decora-tions in the stores. Olivia usually feels very confident that she can get everything done. She typically spends her time in November planning and preparing for her family's Thanksgiving meal, and it isn't until the first of December that she usually starts to panic about Christmas. In October or November, when Olivia might have time to shop for Christmas gifts, she usually convinces herself that it is too early and that she has plenty of time. There is no reason to worry. As Thanksgiving approaches, she tells herself that she will get it all done the weekend after Thanksgiving, when all the sales will be going on, but more often than not other activities interfere. Olivia's overly optimistic self-talk makes her procrastinate every year. This year, she promised herself it would be different. This year she would go in a different direction and try more realistic self-talk.

Since "don't worry about it" is Olivia's catchphrase, her plan is to listen for it, and when she hears it she will tell herself that this is what she says to avoid having to take action right away. Here is her plan. First, in her mind, Olivia will say, "Don't worry about it? Yeah, right! That's what you always say." Second, she will remind herself that this expression is just a way to allow herself to procrastinate. Third, she will remind herself of how stressful it is to scramble at the last minute to get things done during the holidays. Fourth, she will tell herself, "Even if you have plenty of time, it always helps to get a few things done ahead of time." In this way she is not trying to talk herself out of the idea that there is time. Instead, she is telling herself that this does not mean she can't do a few things early.

## How to Get Organized

Most people figure out how to get organized by experimenting or by observing other organized people. Some people seem to be naturally more organized than others. It may be because they had highly organized role models when growing up or because that is just how their brains work. My parents seemed pretty organized. I'm fairly organized, and so are my children. However, each of us has our areas of complete disorganization as well. Here are some steps you can take to get organized if it doesn't seem to come naturally to you.

### Pick a Task

There are many ways to get organized, but the first step is always to pick a task to do. Most of the time this is a simple procedure. We have assigned tasks that have real deadlines, like turning in a paper by the last day of class, paying the rent by the first of the month, filing taxes by April 15th, or buying gifts by Christmas Day. It is easier when there is a set deadline, but unfortunately most of what we do has no such deadline, so it is harder to decide what to do first or when to get started.

Not knowing where to start can make you feel overwhelmed, and that overwhelmed feeling can stop you before you start. If you are tired of spinning your wheels, try Changing Directions 9. It was designed to help you pick a task by focusing on short-term goals—things that need to be done within the next week. You can use a similar strategy for long-term goal planning, but the purpose of this exercise is to help you maneuver around roadblocks in completing day-to-day tasks. Give it a try and start heading in the right direction.

---

↺ Changing Directions 9
## Finding Your Focus

1. **Make a list.** At the beginning of each week, make a list of the things you need to accomplish during the week. Do not include tasks that are easy to do or that you do automatically, like brushing your teeth or going to work or school. You can make the list on a piece of paper, a sticky note, a computer file, a diary, or a marker board. The list needs to be something that you can see throughout your day.

2. **Include deadlines.** If there is a real deadline for completing the task, write the deadline next to the item. Some people like putting the list in order of importance, but that is not necessary at this point.

3. **Keep it simple.** Limit the list to no more than five tasks. If you have more than five on your list, cross off the things that can be delayed or that are not high in importance. You can always add more items to the list as you accomplish the others, but avoid having more than five tasks on your list at any one point in time. If five seems overwhelming to you, limit the list to three items and pick those that need to be done in the first part of the week.

---

4. **Delete and go.** As tasks are completed, erase them from the list. Some people like to keep the list and cross off items as they are finished so they can see what they've accomplished. If that is what you prefer, cross the items off and review the list for a day or two. After that, permanently delete the items from your list.

5. **Pay attention.** Learn from the experience. It is hard to know how many items to put on the list until you have a sense of what you can accomplish. If you find that there are always two tasks you have not completed by the end of the week, you are including too many items on the list.

### ✑ A Personal Note

*I keep a marker board on the wall next to my desk. Each Monday when I come in to work, I make a list of the tasks I would like to get done during the week. I have more to do than can fit on the marker board, but to keep myself focused, I keep only five items on my to-do list on the board and I erase items as they are completed. A short list seems manageable even though I know there are dozens of other things that also need to be done. Today the list includes: edit Chapter 4, make airplane reservations, buy dog food, grade exams, finish data analysis.*

Arthur's weekly list includes the names of three clients whose tax returns must be completed this week. He also added a reminder to finish the budget report for the support group and to buy more shampoo at the store. Bob's list includes getting the oil changed in his car, buying a birthday gift for his daughter, mailing the gift to his daughter, and making an appointment with his dentist. Evelyn's list includes paying her dorm fees, calling her cell phone company to increase her minutes, doing a load of laundry, and making a cake for her friend's birthday. Each had many other things to accomplish, but these items were considered high priority and high importance.

Olivia decided to try this strategy during the Christmas season. Starting in October, she made a very short holiday to-do list every week. In the first few weeks she tried to do too much, which started to cause her more stress. She reminded herself that the holiday season was supposed to be fun and she didn't want her efforts to stop procrastinating to make her a nervous wreck. She figured out how to adjust her list with a smaller number of activities that could be done in just a few hours each week, such as buying Christmas cards and stamps and finding the address list she set up on her computer last year. She used sticky notes with a Christmas design for this special to-do list and stuck the list to her computer screen. When she finished the list, she threw it away and started on a new one. She did not stick to a strict weekly schedule, because sometimes the items on her list took less time and sometimes they took more time. She liked the feeling that went with tearing up the note sheet and throwing it away rather than crossing items off. This strategy helped Olivia get an earlier than usual start on her Christmas tasks.

## Set Priorities

If you have a complicated life that includes work, school, a social life, or a family, you can find yourself with several deadlines hanging over your head at one time. For example, Freddie goes to college, works part-time, and has his own apartment and a dog to take care of. In any given week he may need to finish homework, cover for someone at work, do laundry, take his dog out for a walk, and pay his bills. Sometimes there are not enough hours in the week for it all. In fact, you too will probably conclude that you don't have enough time if you list every task you have to do. This is especially likely if you have high standards for the end product of your efforts. Getting organized means setting priorities.

Prioritizing has two components:

1. *How important is the task?* The first component is to put your responsibilities in some order of importance. Importance can be defined in the following ways:

- There is a real deadline for finishing the task.
- There will be negative consequences for not getting it done.
- It is highly important to you.
- It is highly important to a loved one.
- It will help you succeed.
- It will make your life easier.

Write down your priorities in order of importance with the most important thing you have to do listed first.

2. *How high does the quality of your performance need to be?* The second step in prioritizing is to decide on the quality of performance needed from you. For example, you may have people coming to your home for a visit at the end of the week. Your priority may be to clean up the house before they arrive. The quality required may be low if the people are not picky about the environment and care more about visiting with you than about whether or not you vacuumed the carpet. The quality might need to be high if you are trying to impress someone or avoid criticism. Consider the following factors when deciding the level of quality that each task requires. They are organized from lowest to highest with regard to the quality required in completing the task.

- *If I did at least part of the task, it would be an improvement.*
- *No one cares how well it is done. People care only that an effort was made.*
- *It is only a first try. I can fix it up later, or others can work on it too.*
- *It is more important to have something accomplished than to have it done perfectly.*
- *It would be better for the quality to be high, but no one will fuss if it is fair.*
- *It requires an excellent effort, but it is OK if it is not perfect.*
- *It must be done perfectly.*

For the items you have put on your priority list, rate the level of quality needed for each on a scale from 1 to 10 with 10 being the highest level of quality required (i.e., perfection) and 1 being the lowest level of quality. This may not be easy for complex tasks or if you have a belief or style that makes you reflexively give high or low ratings. For example, Olivia is a perfectionist by nature, so she tends to overrate the level of quality needed by rating all tasks as 10s. This makes everything seem like a high priority and overwhelms Olivia. Freddie, on the other hand, is a bit of a slob, and so he tends to rate the quality required for most things as low. He tends to invest the minimal effort, but that works for him. Dorothea rates picking the right color for her living room paint as a 10 and the clean-up after the work is done as a 10, but the quality needed for the actual painting is only a 7. She is renting the apartment, so she is not very particular about the walls. Bob rated getting his daughter just the right gift as a 10 and is willing to spend a lot of time on it. In contrast, everything else is a 2 or 3.

With both pieces of information—importance and quality required—you can better organize your week. There is no magic formula for rating each item. In general, the more important tasks should be tackled first. If the others are not completed or if only partial progress is made, there will be fewer consequences than for missing a top-priority activity. Tasks that require a high level of quality might not be urgent but are likely to be time consuming. You will have to schedule a larger block of time to get them done. The purpose of these ratings is to make you think about the realistic limitations on time and energy in relation to the amount of time and energy needed to complete your tasks. Planning ahead will decrease the chance that you will procrastinate.

By Thanksgiving, Olivia was more prepared than usual for Christmas, but she still had more to do than there seemed to be time available to complete. She was trying to set more realistic goals this holiday season, but there were still many things she wanted to do for her family, friends, neighbors, and church. Usually she tried to do it all and either stressed herself out trying to get them done or did less and felt awful about it. Knowing this pattern and feeling motivated to improve, Olivia decided to try prioritizing her plans. She hoped that by taking on the most important tasks first, she would not feel as bad if the smaller and less important ones were neglected. Here is her list:

| Olivia's Priority List for December | | |
|---|---|---|
| Task | How Important? | Quality |
| Buy gifts for: | | |
|    Best friend | Very | High |
|    Church pastor | Kind of | Moderate |
|    Mail carrier | Optional | Low |
|    Newspaper delivery person | Optional | Low |
|    Neighbor's kid | Optional | Low |
| Mail the gifts | Very, very | Low |
| Bake five different types of cookies | Not very | Very high |
| Get new ornaments for tree | Not at all | High |
| Host a party for coworkers | Somewhat | High |
| Prepare Christmas dinner | Extremely | Very high |

Olivia revised the list a few times before she felt comfortable with it. Her plan was to put most of her time and energy into the things that were the highest priority. She decided that if the importance was low or the task was optional, she would do those last. In fact, she dropped them from her priority list and created a separate list of things to do if she found herself with extra time. Prioritizing felt good to Olivia because it gave her permission not to do the optional tasks rather than feeling guilty when she ran out of time and didn't get to them.

## ✑ *A Personal Note*

*My husband and I are selling our home and moving to a smaller one now that our sons have grown up and moved out on their own. It seems like there are a hundred things to get done in preparation for this move. They are all important. None of them are fun to do. All of them take time that we do not have at the moment. In addition to the house stuff, I have two classes to teach, exams to grade, and a big grant to write that is due at about the time we will be moving into our new home. Right now, it seems pretty impossible that all of the deadlines will be met.*

*I also have a list of things I would like to do before we move. I would really like the closets to be cleaned out so that I do not pack and move junk from my old closets to my new closets. We have lived in this house for 16 years and have accumulated lots of clutter. I would like my current house to look especially clean and shiny before potential buyers start looking at it. It seems to me that first impressions count, and a shiny kitchen floor might distract them from other things in the house that are less than perfect. I would like to clear out the old clothes that no one wears anymore, including the clothes I am holding on to in hope of losing weight. I have had them in the closet for four years now, and there are no signs that my waistline will be shrinking anytime soon. It would be great if I had time to get my garage better organized before the move so that when we move to a new garage everything will be clean, neatly organized, and labeled. I would also like to get back on my exercise program because everything seems to go better when I am in better shape.*

*It is pretty obvious that all of these things will not get accomplished, as I would prefer. I have done a reality check, and I hold no fantasies that my days will lengthen by several hours or that my energy will be greater than it is now or that someone else will take over my responsibilities. Getting my head out of the clouds and knowing the realities helps me plan. Today I will write until I can't write anymore. I will then work on my closets until I run out of steam or get bored with it. Knowing myself, I will need a time of rest, and then I can do a little more just before bedtime. Today I do not have time to procrastinate. I can accept that because I know that my efforts will all be worth it in the long run.*

## Plan Your Schedule

Another practical skill that can help you get out of the habit of pro-crastinating is to learn to manage your time. There are five things that can help:

1. Assess your available time and energy.
2. Avoid underestimating how long it takes to get things done.
3. Avoid overestimating how much you can get done with the time you have.
4. Match your goals and plans to your schedule.
5. Reassess your goals and make adjustments as needed.

The best way to avoid overestimating how much you can get done and underestimating how much time a task will take is to gather information about the task and look closely at your schedule. You can estimate how long a task will take to complete based on your prior experience or by asking others for their opinions. Remember to add to the estimate the extra time you will need to gather your supplies together, get organized, go to the place where your task must be done, and then finish and put your materials or tools away. The task itself can be a quick one, but you add to the time if you have to go to another location or if any preparation work must be done first. Once you have a more realistic estimate of time, look at your schedule and figure out specifically when you would do the work. For example, if you are thinking about doing something after work, consider how much time you will have after you drive home, eat dinner, or do all the other things you usually do after work.

One of the tools that can prevent you from taking on more than you can handle at any given time is a scheduling program on your computer or a calendar or day planner. When you take on a task, block out the time needed to do it. When you run out of open slots, it means you can't possibly do anything else. If you have a tendency to overestimate how much you can do with the time you have and you know you will have days when you won't get much done, always add 10 or 15% more time to your estimate.

Dorothea defeats herself before she even gets started. She procrastinates for so long that her options for dealing with a problem are reduced. She has wanted to paint her living room for almost a year. Her father helped her move in but has not seen the place since then. He is a perfectionist. He noticed how dirty and dingy the walls looked when he moved her in, and he will notice when he returns that she has not done anything about it. She could have taken her time and painted more slowly. She could have painted when she had some time off from work. She could have hired someone to do it. She could have taken her friends up on their offers to help her. She did none of that because she wanted to do it herself. It did not seem like an overwhelming task. Now that she has waited until the last few weeks before her father returns, she has to get the room painted quickly or not paint it at all and let her dad see her lack of progress.

Not wanting to see the disappointment in her father's eyes, Dorothea decided to paint the room. She tried to find a professional painter to do it for her but could not find someone who could get it done on her time schedule. She knew she would have to do it herself. Dorothea's plan was to paint one wall per night for four nights. She allowed a fifth day for drying and would clean up the mess on day six. If she had started the prior week as planned, she would have had five days to spare before her father arrived.

While on the surface Dorothea's plan seemed reasonable, it did not account for the rest of her schedule and her available energy. She went to work at 8:00 A.M. and usually did not get off until about 6:00 or 6:30 P.M. Her job could be exhausting at times. When she left work, she usually didn't want to do more than have dinner and sit on the couch. Even feeding her cat sometimes seemed like more than she could handle. This week she had a special project to do at work that would demand more of her time and energy. At the end of her workday she would be physically spent. No energy would be left for painting. When Dorothea made her painting plan, she had not considered how she would feel when she got home. Her plan was unrealistic, and when it failed, it only made her feel worse.

It would be easy to say that Dorothea's real problem is that she waited a year to paint her living room. We could argue that she should not have put it off for so long. She should have asked for help sooner. She would not disagree with these statements. In fact, she tells herself these things all the time. The problem is that getting angry with herself, ruminating over her regrets, and thinking about what she should have done or could have done does not help her cope with the painting problem. She needs a strategy for setting goals and expectations that can be more realistically accomplished.

Dorothea has picked the task she thinks is important. She has estimated the time it will take to get it done. She has to realistically evaluate her schedule and make it all fit. After giving it a lot of thought and considering how she usually feels at the end of her workday, Dorothea decided to take two days off from work to paint her living room. Work is light at the moment, and having a freshly painted room is worth using a few vacation days. There is more painting to do than can realistically be done before her father arrives, so she considers allowing him to help her paint the wood trim and doors when he visits. He will enjoy helping, and it is always fun for her to work alongside him.

Poor time management was a big problem for Olivia as well. That was why she got behind on shopping or had to scramble at the last minute and settle for gift cards instead of real gifts. It never before had occurred to her that she consistently underestimated how much time Christmas shopping took. When she thought about it, she realized how many times she had planned to get all her shopping done the weekend after Thanksgiving and how rarely she had been able to accomplish this. This time Olivia estimated that each gift would take approximately 45 minutes to buy if she counted travel time to the mall and between stores. If she had four more gifts to buy, she would need three hours unless she got and found all the items in one store. With this estimate in mind, she was able to schedule her shopping trips so that she had sufficient time to get everything done.

## Avoid Distractions

Tracy can do all the exercises described in this chapter and still fail to overcome her procrastination. She can prioritize her responsibilities, pick the optimal time of day to take on jobs she has been avoiding, and still not get anything done. In her heart of hearts Tracy doesn't really want to do the tasks she has been avoiding. They are difficult, tedious, and not enjoyable. It does not take much to throw her off course. The most common distraction is her telephone. Tracy has a big family and lots of friends. It seems that during her free time her phone rings nonstop. Tracy tells herself that it would be rude to let a call go to voice mail when she could easily answer it, so she stops what she is doing to take every call.

Another distraction for Tracy is her television. When it comes to procrastinating on household chores, Tracy thinks it is less painful to do chores if the television is on. While there is some logic to this idea, the plan doesn't work for Tracy because she finds herself getting engrossed in a movie and ignoring her chores altogether. When you don't really want to do a task, it is easy to allow yourself to get distracted from it. Check out the Shortcuts for Avoiding Distractions that follow. Be honest with yourself and create a work environment where distractions are less likely to occur.

▶▶❙ Shortcuts for
**Avoiding Distractions**

Think about which distractions are most likely to occur and do your best to ignore them or to avoid them. The following might be helpful tactics:

- Turn off the TV if it will distract you from your task.

- Turn off your phone or allow calls to go to voice mail while you are doing your chore.

- Put a "Do Not Disturb" sign on your door to keep out unwelcome visitors.

- Work for short periods of time, only for as long as your attention span will last.

- Use headphones to block out distracting noises.

- Work in an environment with fewer distractions, such as a library.

- Announce to others that you are about to do a chore and do not want to be disturbed.

- When you become aware of a distraction, tell yourself to ignore it.

- When your mind becomes distracted with other things you must do, tell yourself that you can do only one thing at a time.

- When you get distracted, try to come back to your task as quickly as possible.

- If thoughts of more enjoyable activities distract you, tell yourself to stop, focus, and finish what you are doing.

The shopping mall was full of distractions during the holidays, especially if Olivia shopped with her best friend. They would set out with a list of gifts to buy and end up finding great sales on things for themselves. Trying on new outfits, stopping for lunch, and shopping for shoes filled their day. While outings like these were a great deal of fun, they did not always result in Olivia's finishing her Christmas shopping. If Olivia wanted to avoid distractions, she was going to have to shop alone for the things she really needed and schedule a separate shopping trip with her friend just for fun.

## Take a Step Forward

Once you have zeroed in on what you want to accomplish, you might still have trouble getting started on it. My students have trouble getting started on the term papers they write for my class. They think they have to start at the beginning of the paper and work to the end. They can get stuck on the first sentence or the first paragraph and not go any further. No one said they had to start at the beginning, but many have gotten the idea during their education that they have to write straight through from the first sentence to the last sentence. The same can be true for any task. Although there are many ways to get most tasks done, some people think they have to start at the beginning, wherever that seems to be. If you can't figure out where to start, you might procrastinate until you can figure it out.

Sarah is smart and capable, but she gets stuck because she is never really certain where or how to get started. Sarah will procrastinate until her stress over not getting started is so huge that she just impulsively takes action and tells herself, "I don't care if it is the right thing; I just need to get it done." Sarah did this a lot when she was going to school. If she had to do a project or write a report, she would not know how to start. So she wouldn't start. She wouldn't even plan a way to start. She would get so overwhelmed with the idea of making the wrong choice that she would just shut down and make no choice. When time would nearly run out before her report was due, she would switch from fear to determination. Her friends would hear her say, "I don't care anymore. I don't care if it is wrong. I don't care if it turns out badly. If the teacher doesn't like it, that's her problem." With this shift in mind-set came a change in emotions. She felt bold, free of fear, and almost defiant. She would charge through the project, and in most cases she got a fairly good grade.

Sarah needed that attitude shift to get her unstuck from her procrastination. Although her shift from fear to courage was not planned or executed intentionally, it worked. Too bad Sarah could not find her way to that courage a little earlier and save herself weeks of stress.

In the next box are some Shortcuts for getting started when you feel stuck in the mud and you are spinning your wheels.

⸻

▶▶ Shortcuts for
## Getting Started

- **Talk it over before you start.** When you are stuck before you start, rather than procrastinate, talk with others about it. While the person you talk to may not always have a good suggestion, there is something about hearing yourself think out loud that can give you a new perspective. You just need to see an open lane and you are on your way.
- **Jump into the middle.** If you are not sure how to get started, don't start at the beginning. Jump into the middle and go back to the beginning after you have done some work. If you are writing a paper for school and can't figure out the opening paragraph, skip it and write a different section. By the time you are ready, the opener will be easier to write. If you have to do a big and overwhelming project like filing your tax return or applying for a job, don't let uncertainty take control. Just start anywhere so that you feel some movement. After a while how to get the project finished will become clearer.
- **Picture the end product.** If you are not sure how to get going on a project, start by thinking of the end product. Ask yourself a few questions, like:

　　—If it all worked out fine, what would the end result look like?
　　—What would be the best outcome?
　　—What do I want to accomplish?

Visualize the end product. Think about how good it would feel if you stopped procrastinating and accomplished your goal.

Another way to start at the end is to think about all the times you handled a situation or problem or project or task or person and it turned out OK. Try to remember the other times when you were not sure where to start, but you were able to handle things even when it might have been difficult or challenging. When your uncertainty about how to begin has you stuck in the mud, get some leverage by listing the times you were successful.

Olivia understood how some people might have trouble getting started. She found that prioritizing her list of things to do in preparation for Christmas made it easier to figure out where to start. When it came to other things, Olivia could get stuck before she got started. For example, she decided to try scrapbooking. She saw several examples of scrapbooks at a party she had recently attended. She had drawers full of photographs that she had always intended to organize. If she had to organize hundreds of photographs to find the right ones for her project, she would never get it done. In fact, she felt so overwhelmed with the prospect of doing this that she gave up on the project and put the supplies in the drawer along with the photos.

Six months passed before she considered scrapbooking again. Her niece was getting married, and Olivia wanted to give her a scrapbook of pictures that she had collected. The wedding was a year away, so there was plenty of time to get it done. As soon as Olivia heard herself say this, she realized that this was her way of procrastinating again. When she asked herself why she was procrastinating on something that would be enjoyable to do, she had to admit to herself that it was because she didn't want to have to start with reorganizing the photos. Starting at what she thought was the beginning would be too hard, even if she had a year to do it.

Olivia's sister, the mother of her bride-to-be niece, was much more organized about photos than Olivia was, so she decided to ask her for her help in creating the scrapbook. They came up with a two-step plan. First, Olivia and her sister would get together one evening for wine, pizza, and their favorite chick flick. They would eat, drink, watch, and sort through photos with the goal being to pick out photos of Olivia's niece for the scrapbook. The rest of the photos would just go back into their boxes. Olivia and her sister are multitaskers, and since they had seen the movie at least four other times together, it did not need their undivided attention. Making it a social event helped to get Olivia started on her project. Getting help from her sister transformed it from something difficult and unpleasant to something enjoyable. The decision to take out only the photos she needed and leave the rest in their disorganized state made the task more manageable.

You have managed to make it through nearly half of this book, and you have accomplished quite a few things. You have begun to understand why you procrastinate. You have also learned how your negative thoughts and stressful emotions can fuel your tendency to procrastinate and how controlling those thoughts and feelings can help you cope more actively. You have figured out that by changing some of your actions, like getting more organized, setting priorities, and avoiding distractions, you don't have to rely on procrastination as your only way to cope when things get stressful.

Some procrastinators hesitate because they doubt themselves and their abilities. They fear making mistakes, so they put things off until they absolutely have to take action. The next chapter offers suggestions for how to deal with fear of failure and self-doubt. It builds on the strategies you have already learned for controlling negative thinking and for approaching tasks one step at a time. If you've ever hesitated because of self-doubt, Chapter 5 will help you gain more self-confidence.

## The Procrastinators Support Group Pledge Revisited

You may recall from Chapter 1 that the Procrastinators Support Group members recite their pledge at the beginning of each meeting. It helps put them in the right frame of mind for making changes in their behavior. Take a minute and ask yourself if you are ready to take the pledge.

*"I am a person who sometimes chooses to put things off for a while.*

*"I usually have a good reason, even if I am not fully aware of it.*

*"I have to admit that procrastination works for me some of the time, but I want to change.*

*"I can learn to do things differently."*

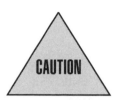

The forces that make you procrastinate are still present. These forces include powerful ideas and feelings that can pull you off your path to progress and back onto the road to procrastination. If you want to change, you have to be strong. You have to believe in your ability to be better tomorrow than you are today. Remember the last line of the pledge: *"I can learn to do things differently."*

# 5 Moving from Self-Doubt to Self-Confidence

**Directions:**

START: Learn about the power of words.

⟹ Begin to respond to your inner child with encouraging thoughts.

⟹ Confront your fear of failure.

⟹ Listen to your inner coach.

END: Let your self-confidence help you take action.

## How Self-Doubt Can Make You Procrastinate

Self-doubt was the topic of discussion at the recent Procrastinators Support Group meeting. Denise, a lifelong self-doubter, told the group about the trouble she had been having in dealing with her landlord. She did not have the confidence to be direct with him when he threatened to raise her rent, so she procrastinated in talking to him until it was too late to negotiate a new lease. She had to move out.

"I know where you're coming from, Denise. I've put myself in the same situation. I kick myself later for being such a chicken," admitted Sarah.

Sometimes Denise's uncertainty and self-doubt caused her to put things off for so long that the problem was handled by someone else. Sometimes the problem would be resolved on its own, and at times she could procrastinate for so long that the problem could be forgotten and ignored. Denise considered these good outcomes. Passively coping in these ways lifted the burden from her. When that happened, Denise could convince herself that she was not responsible for the outcome and therefore could not be criticized or blamed.

As you might expect, there is a downside for people like Denise, who cope in such a passive manner. When someone else handles your problem, he or she may not do a very good job of it or may resolve it in a way you don't like. When you neglect a problem until it resolves itself, the resolution can be a bad one, as with Denise's apartment.

Sarah joined the group's discussion by sharing how her procrastination with the phone company had cost her a lot of money. "Last month I needed to talk to the phone company about some long-distance phone charges I had on my phone bill that were errors," she started. "I wasn't sure what to say to the phone company, and I didn't think the phone company would believe me and delete those charges. So I just paid the bill to make the problem go away," she finished with a look of shame on her face.

For Denise and Sarah, doubt in their abilities to handle problems led them both to procrastinate and, in some cases, to avoid solving important problems. Does lack of confidence make you procrastinate even when the consequences are high? Do you talk yourself out of taking action, even when you know what to do? If so, this chapter provides some guidelines for working around your self-doubt and getting on track to solve problems and make decisions. Learn more about the situations in which self-doubt could be at the root of procrastination.

## The Power of Words

If you have ever been offended by the harsh remarks of someone attacking you, or motivated by an encouraging speech from your coach, or brought to tears by the poignant message of an emotional speaker, you understand the power of words. Your own words can affect your heart and mind the same way words impact you when they come from other people. When you say things to yourself such as "I can't do it" or "It's not going to work," these statements can become instantly believable, override your logic, and weaken your determination.

As you learned in Chapter 3, negative self-talk can shut you down before you have a chance to get started. The negative words that cause you to procrastinate are usually exaggerated or inaccurate, but that does not keep them from zapping your motivation and lowering your self-confidence. The following box contains a list of common negative self-statements that can fuel your doubt and make you procrastinate, even when it is important not to hesitate. Do any of them sound familiar to you? When you read through the list, take notice of what happens to your feelings of motivation. These thoughts are so discouraging that they could even stop a workaholic in her tracks.

## Thoughts That Can Fuel Your Self-Doubt

- "I can't do it; I can't handle it."
- "It's going to be too hard."
- "I don't know what to do."
- "I'm going to mess it up."
- "It's not going to work."
- "It will put me in a bad mood."
- "I can't do it by myself."
- "I'm too tired."
- "I'm not smart enough."
- "No one is going to listen to me."
- "I messed it up last time."

You can learn to cope with thoughts that make you doubt yourself. Throughout this chapter are various strategies that teach you to cope by learning to talk back to your negative self-talk or to analyze your thinking and work through these mental roadblocks that make you procrastinate. Changing Directions 10 focuses on responding to the kinds of thoughts listed in the box by addressing them the way a parent might address a child's resistant words.

---

↺ Changing Directions 10

## Quiet Your Inner Child

Your negative thoughts (like the ones listed in the preceding box) are similar to the excuses given by children who don't want to do their homework. When a child says, "I don't wanna. I'm too tired. I don't know how," most adults respond by challenging those ideas. Mom says, "I don't care if you don't wanna. You have to do it anyway." Dad says, "You're too tired? You weren't too tired a minute ago when you were playing." Teachers say, "If you don't know how, read the directions or ask for help." None of them hear the excuses of children as facts. Your discouraging thoughts that make you put things off are the voice of your inner child. You have to be the grown-up and talk to it like you would talk to a child who is making excuses. Here are some examples:

| Discouraging Thoughts of Your Inner Child | Your Grown-Up Responses |
| --- | --- |
| *"I can't handle it."* | *"I always say that when I'm stressed."* |
| *"I don't know what to do."* | *"Slow down. Figure it out or ask for help."* |
| *"It's not going to work."* | *"Come up with a plan that is more likely to work."* |

---

## ⊘ *A Personal Note*

*My inner child really likes my bed. In the morning when the alarm goes off, I hit the snooze button automatically, because my inner child doesn't want to get out of bed. My inner child loves my soft blanket and my cushy pillow. My inner child says, "You can still get to work on time. Ten more minutes won't hurt." I listen to my inner child until the grown-up me remembers what waits at work. The grown-up me spoils the moment by reminding me that if I don't get up now, I will probably not have time for breakfast. The grown-up me remembers that I have an early morning meeting and that I have to dress like a grown-up for it. That means I need the extra time to get ready. My inner child rolls over and tells my husband, "You shower first. I need five more minutes." He ignores me, because his inner child likes the bed too.*

# Substitute Motivating Statements for Self-Defeating Statements

You might remember from Chapter 1 that a major reason you procrastinate is that you can often get away with it. Consequences do not always follow procrastination. Things eventually work themselves out, or you suffer the negative consequences and get over them in time. The main reason you can get away with procrastination is that you eventually take action even if it is at the last minute. When your anxiety over not getting something done gets more intense than your urge to procrastinate, you get into gear. Your mind switches from procrastination-enhancing thoughts to motivating, butt-kicking, panicking thoughts like "I've got to get this done now!"

One way to stave off the urge to procrastinate is to call those motivating thoughts to mind earlier, *before* you have to panic. You can activate your inner butt-kicker before your situation reaches a crisis level. The next box includes some examples of motivating self-talk. These are the ideas that usually come to mind when people are about to suffer a consequence for their procrastination. They are what we tell ourselves when there's absolutely no more room for delay. Add yours to the list and then put reminders of these motivational statements where you are likely to need them—in the places you're likely to go when you procrastinate, such as on a sticky note near your computer or television or video game unit. Or write the statements that sound like your inner butt-kicker on an index card and carry them around with you or type them into your screen saver so that you see them whenever you are in front of your computer. The idea is simply to expose yourself to these motivating beliefs before the fear of a serious consequence exerts its own motivation—at the very last minute.

## Motivating Statements

- "I have to do it now or I'm going to get in trouble."
- "It absolutely has to be done."
- "I'm doing it now no matter what."
- "I don't care what else has to be done."
- "Everything else will have to wait."
- "Stop making excuses."
- "I'm not going to make it unless I work all night."
- "I don't have a choice."
- "Don't be a loser."
- "Get off your butt and do it."
- "You are out of time."

### ✑ *A Personal Note*

*I was a cheerleader in high school. In fact, I was head varsity cheerleader in my senior year. I cheered for a football team that rarely won a game in the four years I was in high school. Our greatest accomplishment was a tied score with our cross-town rivals. We not only got used to losing; we expected it. It was not a big deal. In fact, we had a tremendous amount of school spirit. There was no pressure to win championships.*

*Every week we had pep rallies with cheering and dancing and speeches from the players and coaches. We had a wonderful time. We made up slogans to put on posters that showed our belief in our team's abilities, our pride in our school, and our excitement about another Friday night under the lights. We approached every game with the belief that it might be possible to win.*

*I learned a great deal about life during those years. I got good at cheering on efforts even when the odds were against us. I learned how to sustain hope when others gave up. I could conquer doubt because it was more fun to be encouraging than to be discouraging. Maybe that is why I always feel hopeful when a new patient comes to my office, even when that person has suffered hardships or feels discouraged or hopeless.*

*When I have had personal troubles in life, it is a little harder to get in touch with my inner cheerleader. I have to catch myself thinking discouraging thoughts and mentally put on my uniform. (In my mind it still fits.) It would be great if there were a squad of screaming fans behind me, but there is just me. It's a good thing I know how to rally my own spirit. Here is how I do it. I think back on the times that others had doubt and I believed. I remember the times that were hard and painful but still turned out for the best. I know that I can recover from hardship because I have done it before. I know that even though it would be easier to procrastinate, I will enjoy the feeling of accomplishment when my task is done. I just have to pick up the megaphone in my mind and yell, "Come on, Basco. Let's go!!"*

▶▶ Shortcuts for
## Accessing Your Inner Cheerleader

1. Has there ever been a time when others had doubt but you had faith? What words of encouragement would

you have offered at that time? (*"You can do it!" "Don't give up."*)

2. Try to remember a painful time that you thought would never end. Find a word or two that describes how it felt when it was over. (*"Victorious." "I'm a survivor."*)

3. Call to mind one hardship that you have been through in the past. Think of a word or two that describe what you did to get through it. (*"Fought." "Hung in there."*)

4. When was the last time you felt a sense of accomplishment? Pick a word or two to describe how that felt. (*"Relief." "Peaceful." "Successful."*)

5. Think of a positive and self-affirming phrase that you believe when you are in good spirits. (*"I'm smart and capable." "I can handle it."*)

6. Name one or two things about yourself that make you think you can ultimately succeed. (*"I don't easily give up." "I can usually figure things out."*)

7. Create in your mind a slogan that could cheer you on when you are feeling discouraged. (*"Go for it and be victorious." "You can make it happen!"*)

**GO, FIGHT, WIN!**

## Face the Fear of Making a Big Mistake

Bob was separated from his wife for four years before he finally filed for divorce. He was pretty sure their marriage was not going to work out even before she kicked him out, but he hesitated to make the split permanent. When he thought of divorce, a little voice in his head would question him: "What if this is not the right thing to do? What if it was your fault that the marriage didn't work? Maybe you should try again. What if you never find anyone else and you are alone for the rest of your life?" These doubts would plague him until he had another disagreement with his wife that showed she was never going to change and he could never live with her again. It went back and forth like this year after year. Staying married was better for his wife, who was still on Bob's health insurance plan, drove his car, and lived in their house. Bob stayed in the marriage because he was afraid of making a mistake. He doubted his ability to make this decision and feared that if it were a mistake he would regret it for the rest of his life. This may sound melodramatic, but Bob didn't want any more regrets.

Bob could drive himself crazy with his doubts and worries. He imagined loneliness forever without his wife. He pictured himself ill and imagined that no one would help him. His imagination could run wild with the possibilities. When he would get on a roll, he could spend hours running through a number of sad and painful scenarios. His stress would climb. He would give himself a headache as he came to believe that what he imagined would come to pass.

Do you stress yourself out by imagining bad outcomes if you take action? Are you like Bob? Instead of imagining disaster, you need to learn to objectively evaluate the likelihood of a bad outcome and make a decision based on the facts. Changing Directions 11 will walk you through the four steps for counteracting the self-doubt that keeps you from taking action.

---

↻ Changing Directions 11
## Confront Your Fear of Making Mistakes

**Focus:** *Fear of making a mistake*—Your anxiety about taking the wrong action leads you to procrastinate. The fear is that you will make the wrong decision and things will turn out badly.

**Thinking Error:** *Self-doubt*—Not believing in your ability to make a good choice. Focusing on what you could do wrong rather than what could go right.

> **Goal**: Stop jumping to conclusions and scaring yourself into believing that your actions will lead to a bad outcome.
>
> **Step 1**: **Name your fear**. What are you afraid will happen if you stop procrastinating and start taking action? Write down what you imagine. If you are not certain what to write, try to picture in your mind what action you seem to be avoiding. Then ask yourself, "What is the worst thing that can happen?" It is OK if the thoughts you write down seem silly or unrealistic. Most scary thoughts are based more on fear than on fact.

Bob was afraid that if he divorced his wife, he would be missing an opportunity to fix the relationship. He was also afraid that since he was getting older, no one else would want him. He knew that he was hard to live with and that it would take someone special to put up with his quirks. He saw himself alone with only his dog to keep him company. The idea was depressing.

> **Step 2**: **Get the facts**. What makes you think your fear will come true? Make a list of reasons that your action could really have a bad outcome. Try to base this list on facts, not just on fear.

In Bob's case, he was getting older, and it was true that he might not be able to find another suitable spouse. He knew that he was not as attractive as a lot of men. He didn't drive an expensive car or have a lot of nice clothes. Another reason he held off getting a divorce was that there had been a time when he got along well with his wife. He knew that people could change so he held on to this dream for a long time. This fantasy about working things out with his wife was more pleasant than his sad images of loneliness.

> ***Step 3***: **Get real**. What facts would suggest your negative fanta-
> sies would not likely come true? Are there things you are over-
> looking that would guarantee a better outcome?

Bob had a hard time coming up with evidence against his fear
of being alone forever. He knew that he was a nice person with a
"great personality," but he knew he was no Matt Damon or Brad
Pitt or even Harrison Ford. He thought that those were the only
guys that were getting the girls. What Bob needed to help him get
real were some examples of guys like him who seemed to be able to
attract women. When he looked around the room at the support
group members, he noticed that Polly always seemed to pay attention to Arthur. Arthur was Bob's age and not any better looking
than Bob. So maybe that was evidence that average guys could get
a date. Not everyone was alone. Bob also remembered that Polly
tried to get friendly with him until he told her he wasn't over his
divorce. This could also be evidence against his self-doubt.

> ***Step 4***: **Analyze the facts**. Review the evidence for and against
> your fear that you will be making a big mistake by taking action.
> Try to be objective. Is there reason to believe that your self-
> doubt is making you scare yourself unnecessarily? If so, try to
> rely on your logic and make a decision that makes the most
> sense. Rely less on your emotions to guide you.

When Bob reviewed the facts, it seemed to him that he was
selling himself short. His wife had not been willing to work things
out. It was not all about him or about his failures. Even if he had
committed to staying married, she was not willing to do her part to
mend their relationship. Bob realized that he had been assuming
that she was the last woman in the world who would ever have him
and that without her he was condemned to loneliness. Bob knew
better than that. He had let his fear of making a mistake take con-

trol of the situation. He had to accept that the decision to divorce had been his wife's, and he needed to look after himself and stop mourning the loss of his marriage.

▶▶ Shortcuts for
## Overcoming Self-Doubt

Experiments in taking action are a great way to get real about self-doubt. You test out your negative assumption by doing an experiment that could prove you were wrong. For example, Bob needs some experience with trying to attract a woman. He could start with testing his ability to engage women in conversation. He wouldn't have to go out on a date, and he would not have to tell his ex-wife. He could just call it an experiment.

## Fear of Failure

Claudia's self-doubt is a lot stronger. She is afraid not just of making a big mistake but of total failure. She handles it by avoiding situations that could lead to failure. That includes dating, asking for a raise, and trying to go back to college after being away from school for 10 years. When asked about these things by family and friends, Claudia says she plans to take care of them soon, she's looking into the possibility, or she's working on it. None of these statements are true, and everybody knows it. Claudia has had some bad experiences in life with school, with dating, and with jobs. At the moment, her job is going well. It doesn't pay much, but her employer is happy to have her there. She doesn't date, but she has a lot of friends, so she isn't lonely very often. She is smart and likes to read, and that is a substitute for trying to go back to school. "Why mess up a good thing?" she tells herself, although she doesn't really believe it. Claudia has dreams for the future. She wants an education, a home of her own, and maybe a family. To get those things, she has to make some changes. But why set herself up for the possibility of failure? That is Claudia's dilemma, so she continues to procrastinate on making improvements to her life.

In Claudia's mind, if she made a mistake or failed, it would be horrible and irredeemable. Have you ever put something off for fear of failing? If so, you might be catastrophizing, just like Claudia. Chapter 3 explained that catastrophizing means imagining not just a mistake but a catastrophe. When you look at Claudia's story, it is easy to see that she would have little to lose if she took a chance on dating or taking classes or trying to get a better job. While things might not work out perfectly, her efforts probably would not end in disaster. Claudia's fear of failure is holding her back. The decatastrophizing exercise presented in Changing Directions 6 near the end of Chapter 3 can help Claudia stop scaring herself. If you get carried away by self-doubt and become preoccupied with the possibility of failure, go back to Chapter 3 and work through the same exercise. The possible solutions included asking yourself how likely it is that the worst outcome will occur, considering the possibility that you are using catastrophic thinking as an excuse, and asking yourself what advice you would give to a friend or family member with the same fear.

You can also use Changing Directions 11. For example, Step 1 is to name your fear. Claudia is afraid that if she tries to go back to college she will not be able to handle the coursework and will get poor grades or be forced to drop out. It would break her heart to fail again, and it would be humiliating if others knew about it. She imagines how it would feel to have to tell her family that she could not handle school and would now have to settle for a low-paying job and live in an apartment for the rest of her life.

Step 2 is to get the facts that support your scary thought. Claudia's fear is based on a lot of emotion and a few facts. The last time she was in school, it was not easy for her. She had to study a lot to do as well as the other people in her class. She is older now and not as quick or sharp as kids just finishing high school. She has been away from learning for a long time. These are facts that reinforce her fear.

Step 3 is to get real by looking at the evidence against her vision of failure. What Claudia is overlooking is the fact that she has changed for the better since she was last in college. She is more organized, takes learning seriously, enjoys reading more, and now has no trouble remembering what she read, as she did when she was younger and more easily distracted by everything other than schoolwork. Another way she has changed that would make college easier for her now is that she is no longer distracted with trying to meet guys or make friends and she no longer parties every weekend.

Step 4 is to analyze the facts. Remembering how she has changed helps Claudia calm her scary thoughts. When she weighs these facts along with her fears, it is easier to see that there are plenty of reasons to be hopeful and only a few reasons to be scared.

## Venture Outside Your Comfort Zone

Fear of failure can make it difficult for people to go outside their comfort zone to take even small risks. Tracy, for example, is not at risk of losing her job, but she puts off doing extra projects that could help her get a promotion. She is holding back because she is comfortable with her current position, and it doesn't seem worth it to her to risk failure or to have to go through the discomfort of making an effort and maybe having it backfire on her by making her look stupid. For some time she has been thinking that her procrastination was simply laziness, but after hearing the stories of the other support group members, she has come to realize it has more to do with not wanting to go outside her comfort zone.

When she is asked to do a new project at work where she has to come up with new ideas, she feels anxious and puts it off as long as possible. As the deadline nears, her anxiety gets worse and her desire to avoid the whole thing becomes overwhelming. The time pressure adds to the pressure of the task itself until she finally gives in and does the work. The whole time she is procrastinating she is filling her own thoughts with self-doubt. "What if no one likes my idea? What if they think it's dumb and my boss is convinced that I don't deserve a promotion?"

When she finally makes herself do the work and gets positive feedback for it, Tracy realizes the task was not a big deal after all and if she had gotten to it sooner she would not have had to create a crisis situation for herself. Objectively, Tracy can look at her behavior and realize what she is doing. She is procrastinating because she doesn't like leaving her comfort zone. She lacks self-confidence, and she admits that maybe she is a little bit lazy. The funny thing about it is that Tracy knows she is good at her work. She receives praise from others and has gotten awards, and when there is a new or challenging task at work, people go to her first because of her knowledge and skills. Her self-doubt is irrational but still has the power to make her procrastinate. If Tracy could remember the praise, the awards, and the confidence that others have in her the next time she is faced with a challenge, perhaps she would not procrastinate until the last minute. Going outside her comfort zone and doing more could get her a raise. Check out the Shortcut on giving yourself credit. Maybe it will help you remember your strengths when your mind seems to focus on your fears.

▶▶ Shortcuts for
## Giving Yourself Credit

One quick strategy to steer away from self-doubt is to take a moment to call to mind the times when you took action and things turned out OK. Don't limit your list to just those times when you had a great outcome or a big response from others. Consider the times you didn't fail, no one criticized you, you were not humiliated, and no major mistakes were made, as well as situations when a problem occurred and you were able to handle it. Write them down. Put the list where you can easily find it when your self-doubt creeps back in. Add your accomplishments to the list from time to time.

## Coping with Tunnel Vision

Denise lacks self-confidence just like Tracy. It has been a problem all her life. She is the youngest of five children. She has never been as smart as her oldest sister, Sissy; as talented as her oldest brother, Sam; as cute as her sister Meg; or as confident as her star athlete brother, Jack. She has been protected by her siblings and by her parents all her life. They have been there to help her get through school, find her first job, buy her first car, and move into her first apartment. When she has trouble, one of them is always nearby to give her advice or guidance or encouragement. This all sounds wonderful, but Denise would say that all this love has turned her into a wimp. She is so used to being helped that she has no confidence in her ability to handle life on her own. She doesn't think she can handle stress or disappointment. When she thinks about trying to make it on her own, she fears she won't be able to handle it; she'll freak out, go nuts from the stress, or totally screw it up.

She doesn't want her family to think she is a total baby, so she doesn't voice these worries. They would not take her seriously anyway. Just like Tracy, Denise copes by staying in her comfort zone. When opportunities come her way, she delays making a decision until it is too late and the opportunity has passed her by. She was offered a chance to apply for a new position in her company that would mean a move to another state, away from her family. It would have been a promotion, but she didn't think she could handle it, so she delayed updating her résumé until she had missed the application deadline. "Oh well," she told herself, "I'll try for the next one." Denise was invited to go skiing for the first time with a group of friends. She was not as strong as Jack or as courageous as Sissy, so she avoided committing to the trip until it was too late to book an airline ticket.

When Denise is faced with opportunities to venture outside her comfort zone, doubt floods her mind and she forgets about the numerous times she was able to cope, handle herself in difficult situations, and manage without the aid of her family. This memory lapse is called *tunnel vision*. She sees through a small tunnel all the fearful possibilities that would face her and how she is different from her siblings. What doesn't come to mind are the memories from outside her limited tunnel vision, such as the many times when she made a decision on her own and it turned out well or when she surprised herself by handling a difficult situation without the advice or guidance of her family. Tunnel vision makes a person see the negative things that confirm her fear but miss all the other pieces of information—things outside the tunnel—that would give perspective to her worry. Those are experiences or ideas that are contrary to the worry. The solution for building self-confidence is to fight off the tendency to use tunnel vision as your only way of evaluating your choices. Changing Directions 12 will walk you through the steps for getting out of the tunnel and seeing all the facts before making a decision. Give it a try. If it works, make it a daily practice.

---

↺ Changing Directions 12

## Building Self-Confidence by Getting Out of the Tunnel

**Focus**: *Fear of repeating the past*—Calling to mind past failures, mistakes, errors, and bad luck.

**Thinking Error**: *Tunnel vision*—Focusing your attention and calling to mind bad experiences you have had that give you reasons to continue procrastinating while ignoring or dismissing memories of times when you stopped procrastinating in spite of self-doubt and things turned out OK.

**Goal**: Look outside the tunnel and get the big picture by reviewing not only the reasons to continue procrastinating but also the reasons to trust yourself to take action.

**Note**: This is a written task. You will need paper or a computer to keep notes. You may have to work on this over several days until you have a complete list.

---

*Step 1*: **Narrow the focus**. Describe the situation you are avoiding or the focus of your procrastination. Make a list of the reasons you think it may not be a good idea to go forward with your idea or activity. The list might include bad experiences you have had in the past that make you hesitate to try again. Add things about yourself that take away your comfort or confidence to take action. List any other reasons you are holding yourself back. If you have done this correctly, you should be feeling uncomfortable or anxious as you read through this list.

*Step 2*: **Broaden the focus**. Make a second list of reasons to have faith in yourself and your ability to tackle your procrastination. Think of the times you stopped procrastinating on something that you had doubts about and things turned out OK. Don't just list the times when you had a really good outcome or experience. Think of the times you took action rather than procrastinating and nothing bad happened. Taking action does not always result in a super-positive outcome. For most people, the results are often neutral, not a big deal, or just OK. List those too, because they are outside the negative tunnel of bad memories and fearful thoughts.

If you have done this correctly, you should be feeling pretty good about yourself and your actions. If you see the list and tell yourself that those positive experiences don't matter, then your tunnel vision might be a sign of perfectionism. Go to Chapter 7 and review the section on procrastination and perfectionism.

*Step 3*: **Draw a conclusion**. Look over both lists. Do you have examples in both categories? What do you think the examples mean about your ability to stop procrastinating and take action? Is your self-doubt warranted? Do you need to take any precautions to avoid a bad outcome? Make a plan and take the next step.

# Denise's Example

## Narrow the Focus

*The problem*: "I want to buy a car on my own without my dad or brother helping me make the decision."

*Reasons not to take action*: "I'm afraid I will make the wrong choice and buy a car that turns out to be a lemon. My family will scold me for not asking for advice or allowing them to help. They will make fun of me for getting tricked by a sleazy salesperson into making a bad purchase. I will not be able to live it down until I buy the next car, which will inevitably be chosen by my father or big brother. The reason I am afraid is that this has happened in the past. I bought a used couch that turned out to have some broken springs. I thought I was getting a good deal, but it turned out to be a piece of junk. My parents thought it was 'cute' and told my siblings about it. They thought it was funny. When they visited, they made a big deal about not sitting on the broken couch. It was annoying. I bought a queen-size bed that ended up being too big for my apartment. I had to send it back to the store. I got lots of advice about measuring the room and the bed before buying another one. It was embarrassing. I took a job that turned out to be horrible. My boss was a real jerk and kept hitting on me. I quit after the first month. That led to a mountain of advice from my family and several of their friends who had heard about 'poor Denise's' experience. I hate it when I look stupid to my family, and I'm tired of getting advice on how to be a grown-up."

## Broaden the Focus

Reasons to have faith in yourself: "I have made some good decisions in the past. I chose my apartment, which I love. I chose a college major on my own. I choose my friends. I have ignored my family's advice several times and gone my own way, and it turned out fine, like when I chose to work part-time while going to school. When I had problems with money or with my roommate, I fixed them without telling anyone. I bought several good pieces of furniture that fit my apartment nicely without getting any advice from my mom and dad."

### Draw a Conclusion

"I'm not an idiot. I can make decisions on my own. I know some things about buying a car. *Precautions:* I have done some research on cars. I plan to get a used car, but I will have a mechanic look it over before I buy it. I know how much used cars should cost and I know how much I can afford. If it turns out badly, my family will just have to get over it. I can help by not complaining to them if I run into problems the way I did when I was younger."

## Deal with Discouragement

Sometimes self-doubt comes from having experiences that leave you feeling discouraged. When that happens, it is hard to pick yourself back up and feel motivated to keep trying. Toni's SAT scores, for example, were not as high as she had hoped, and she felt discouraged about getting into a good college. Her discouragement made her procrastinate on filling out college applications, asking her teachers for letters of recommendation, and writing her college essays. She knew the deadlines were nearing, but feeling discouraged about her scores made her lose her motivation to apply to colleges.

Willie felt the same way about starting another diet. He had tried many times to lose weight with little and only temporary success. His feelings of discouragement made him put off getting started on a new plan. Olivia felt discouraged about her ability to find a better job. She was unhappy with her position at the local grocery store and wanted a change, but she heard how hard it was for her friends to find good jobs. She told herself that if they couldn't find decent jobs she wouldn't be able to find one either.

If you have ever felt discouraged, you know how hard it is to overcome that feeling and push yourself to take action. Usually we wait until the feeling lifts; when something good happens, that renews our motivation and lifts our self-doubt. For some people the discouragement never lifts, and they give up on their goals. Rather than wait for an external force to give us the encouragement we need, it would be better if we could lift ourselves up during these times. One strategy is to step back and try to access your inner coach. Your inner coach is that encouraging voice that helps you review your plans and consider the importance of taking action and urges you to consider the possibility that your actions could lead to success. Changing Directions 13 will help your inner coach find her voice.

---

## Ↄ Changing Directions 13
## Listen to Your Inner Coach

If your words are strong enough to make you procrastinate, there is a good chance they can be strong enough to talk you into taking action. Learn to counterbalance the part of you that can be discouraging with encouraging ideas. Think of it as your inner coach. Following are some questions you can pose to yourself to help you get started.

- **What have you got to lose?** You may be right that it will be difficult to achieve your goal, but what do you lose by trying? The only way to find out if you can be successful is to make an effort. If you are procrastinating, you are already losing something important—time—so you might want to use that time instead to go after your goal. Any chance is better than none.
- **What is important to you about this task?** Self-doubt and discouragement can make you lose sight of the importance of your goal. The negative thinking that makes you believe you can't handle a situation or won't succeed is the same negative thinking that makes you tell yourself that the goal was not important after all. Take a minute to think about why you wanted to take action in the first place.

- **Could this be your time to succeed?** Sometimes taking on a new activity is all about the timing. If your discouragement comes from having had a bad experience, consider the possibility that your timing was off. Maybe you were not at your best or, through no fault of yours, obstacles kept you from being successful. Maybe now is the time to try again, because now is your time to succeed.
- **What has changed in your favor?** It is easy to lose hope of accomplishing a goal, especially if you tried in the past and did not feel successful. Think of some reasons to be hopeful that the next time you take action it will be effective. Are you different now? Have the circumstances changed? Is there someone around to help who wasn't there before?

## What If You Are Right?

Sometimes fearful thoughts come true. Things do not always work out the way we want, but that doesn't mean the outcome has to be insurmountable. Plan ahead for how you will cope if it looks like you could be headed for a bad outcome. If your plan of action does not go well, your preparation will pay off because you will have a strategy in place for dealing with the consequences.

Claudia isn't sure what she will do if she can't handle college. She has been away from it for so long that she doesn't remember what she is supposed to do if she gets into trouble. Rather than let her fear make her continue to procrastinate, Claudia decided to create a plan for the possibility of failure. Her first step was to talk to one of the young girls at work who was still in college. It was helpful to talk to someone who has dealt with the fears she will be facing. Claudia came up with two plans. The first plan is that she will not try to go back to college all at once. She will first take an adult education class at the local high school just to get her feet wet. If that goes well, she will take an evening class at the local community college in a subject that she thinks she can handle and that is interesting to her, like a psychology course. Claudia's second plan is for what to do if she does not feel like class is going well. Her friend at work told her to talk to her T.A. first and then talk with her professor about her difficulties. If that doesn't work, the learning centers at most colleges have tutors. She will get herself a tutor. In fact, she thinks she might arrange for a tutor before she even needs one, kind of like a security blanket. As part of her plan, she will find out the dates for withdrawing from classes without penalty. She also decided that she would not tell anyone in her family about school until she was sure she was going to be able to pass the course. She figured that she could handle failure better if no one else knew about it.

Bob had a hard time coming up with a good backup plan if things did not go well with dating. He thought he needed two types of plans, one for seeing if he and his ex-wife could get back together and another for meeting new women. He did not think it was a good idea to try to meet women while he was trying to work it out with his ex-wife, so he decided to start with her. Bob was about 99% sure that his ex-wife was dating someone else and had no interest in getting back with him, but he thought he needed to know for sure so that he would not "What if ...?" himself for eternity. He planned to call her next week and try to set up a time to talk. If that did not work out, he would try his hand at meeting someone new. He did not think he could take rejection from another woman right after being rejected by his ex-wife again, so he decided on a two-week waiting period before making his first move. He decided his plan was to start slowly, just like Claudia. He would start by talking more to women in his group, at work, and in church. He would not try to flirt or anything like that. He would start slowly by just trying to make conversation. If that went well, he would try it again. If no one wanted him, he would find other ways to spend his time. He would not just hide in his apartment and wait until his life was over. He would try to make more of an effort to see his daughter and to visit his mother. He might let his friends at work fix him up as they have offered to do in the past. A blind date is better than doing nothing.

## Who Says You Always Have to Succeed?

Procrastination that stems from self-doubt is based on the assumption that making a mistake or failing will be a horrible experience that must be avoided at all costs. The reality is that making mistakes or failing is a normal human experience that occurs for most of us throughout our lives, beginning in childhood. We are trial-and-error learners. When we fail to grab something that is beyond our reach, we complain until someone gets it for us. Out of childhood failure comes the discovery of new ways to cope. We fail and recover over and over again when we learn to walk, to ride a bike, to drive a stick shift, and to use a new computer or cell phone. Most mistakes are learning experiences. They can hurt a little, but they result in disaster much less often than we think they will. Remember that mistakes can be overcome. The sting of humiliation fades with time. We have the ability to adapt, cope, learn, and start over. Make time to work your way through the exercises in this chapter so that irrational fear does not keep you from your dreams.

Although procrastination hurts you more than others, there are situations in which your procrastination can affect the other people in your life. The next chapter focuses on procrastination and relationships. You will learn a few things about how relationships can help maintain procrastination even when it is viewed as a problem. You might also find out what kinds of messages your procrastination sends to others. The more you know, the more control you will have over your procrastination. Keep going. You are making progress.

# 6 | Procrastination in Relationships

**Directions:**

**START:** Find out if you are using procrastination as a tool, weapon, or shield.

➥ Discover how procrastination is used to express anger.

➥ Figure out if you are using procrastination to gain control over others.

➥ Know if trying to please people is fueling your procrastination.

**END:** Learn new ways to communicate with words instead of your actions.

Procrastination is not just something you do by yourself. It becomes part of your relationships with others. You can use procrastination to communicate your feelings to others. For example, putting off a task that someone else wants you to do is a way of letting him know that you don't want to do it. Procrastination can define your relationships with others, like creating dependency when others do things for you because you keep putting them off. Although procrastination can elicit unwanted reactions from others such as anger or frustration, it can help you get the upper hand in relationships, such as when you procrastinate to control when something gets done. Procrastination can also be the reaction you have when you want to avoid people you find it hard to say no to. Procrastination can be a tool that is used to skillfully manipulate others, a weapon that can be used to fight back when they anger you, and a shield that can protect you from being overwhelmed and on the receiving end of others' disapproval.

The goal of this chapter is to help you understand how procrastination affects and is affected by relationships. The skills that are introduced focus on helping you communicate your thoughts, feelings, or needs more directly so you don't have to rely on your procrastination to speak for you.

## Interpersonal Consequences of Procrastination
### It Makes Others Angry

Carla is not only a world-class procrastinator but an Olympic gold medalist several years running. She thinks she may even hold the record for consecutive gold medals in all procrastinator events—those pertaining to home, work, self, and relationships. Carla attributes her success to her ability to train others to work around her procrastination. She feels no guilt for procrastinating on most things. She is a likable person, so most people cut her slack or work around her schedule. If she is invited to a party, her friends assume she will be at least an hour late and plan accordingly. Her mother and best friend lecture her on her tardiness, but for Carla these criticisms go in one ear and out the other. There have been no real consequences that would make her change her habits. At some level she takes pride in her ability to make others adapt to her procrastination rather than the other way around. That is why she is a gold medalist. She believes that if her procrastination caused a problem she would change.

Recently, Carla suffered her first big consequence for procrastination, and it came from a surprising source. Her college roommate, Melissa, is someone that Carla greatly respects. Recently, Melissa got angry with Carla for procrastinating in helping with Melissa's wedding plans. Carla, Melissa's maid of honor, had dropped the ball on booking a place for Melissa's bachelorette party. Melissa had obviously been holding on to her anger for some time, so when she finally let it out, she criticized Carla for all the times she had been late, all the times she had waited until the last minute to get something done, and for stressing out Melissa and Melissa's mother as they prepared for the wedding. "I'm sorry I asked you to be part of my wedding!" Melissa shouted as she burst into tears of frustration. Carla was stunned. There it was—the consequence she secretly thought would eventually come. It did not come from her supervisor at work. It came from someone she respected even more. In her tirade, Melissa said she was embarrassed for Carla because everyone knew she was a procrastinator and people did not take her seriously. Melissa told Carla it hurt her that she had defended Carla so many times when others called her unmotivated or irresponsible and Carla had rewarded her loyalty by letting her down and stressing her out at the most important time in her life. Carla had been clueless.

The very next day Carla set out to make changes. She knew it would not happen overnight, but she tried her best to stop procrastinating. She started with getting up on time in the morning. She was determined not to start her day already behind schedule. She always seemed to be playing catch-up and was self-conscious about how others looked at her. She wondered, when they laughed casually as she walked in late to work if they were really thinking, "What a loser."

Carla was able to sustain her progress most of the time. She still hated getting out of bed early, but the new Carla heard her friend's disappointed tone in her head. Carla believed she deserved Melissa's criticism, but it hurt her feelings, and it was humiliating. She had not been getting away with her procrastination like she thought. She had only been fooling herself. The consequences were more than just her friend's criticism. Everyone knew what she was really like. That is what motivated her to change.

When Carla told her story at the support group meeting, Bob confronted her, saying, "I knew that would happen."

"You knew what would happen?" asked Carla.

"You always downplayed how your procrastination bothered other people. I figured someone would eventually jump your case for it. You are a sweet kid, so no one was going to get in your face about it, but I figured it would eventually bite you in the butt."

"Geez. Thanks for your support, Bob," Carla replied sarcastically.

"What are you going to do about it?" Arthur asked sheepishly. He agreed with Bob and never liked Carla's sarcastic comments about how she got others to work around her procrastination.

"You too?" Carla said, making more of a statement than a question. "Are you against me too?"

"No, honey," said Polly. "We just want to help you come to terms with your procrastination and how it affects people. Don't get mad. You needed to hear what Melissa had to say even though it hurt. Now let us help you."

## ᛩ A Personal Note

*The fact that people do not openly express anger at your procrastination does not mean they are OK with it. When you agree to do something for another person, most of the time that person is going to find it difficult to take issue with you when you seem to be procrastinating. In addition, most procrastinators are good at coming up with creative explanations for why something was not done on time. The other person doesn't want to embarrass himself by accusing you of procrastination when there may be some other, valid reason for your lack of progress.*

*Trust me, as a college professor I have heard many creative excuses for procrastination over the years. There are the usual excuses like my dog ate my homework, my e-mail is down, my printer broke, I was too sick to write my paper, my car broke down, the books I needed were checked out of the library, my thumb drive broke, or I was in jail. I excuse real emergencies whenever there is a doctor's note. The other excuses leave a bad impression and make me doubt the student the next time he or she misses a deadline. I would much prefer a student admit to procrastination and ask for help with it than make up a lame excuse for turning in late work.*

## Others Come to Expect It

This may not seem like a negative consequence of procrastination, especially if you are like Carla and like it when others adjust to your pace of getting things done. However, another downside of procrastination is that part of their adjustment involves learning not to expect much from you. If you are perceived as a chronic procrastinator, you are taken less seriously than the nonprocrastinators around you. That is because you may inadvertently give the impression that you are irresponsible. That was what happened to Carla: people thought less of her but never shared this with her.

If you are a nice person like Carla and well liked by others, there is a good chance that you have not been called out on your procrastination. You might misinterpret this as meaning that your procrastination is not a problem for others. When this topic came up at the Procrastinators Support Group, it was surprising to find out that procrastinators think badly of other procrastinators. Bob was the first to admit that he thought procrastinators had no excuse for their behavior. He considered it laziness. Arthur was a little more sympathetic, but he admitted that he had used his procrastination to get out of things he didn't want to do and he thought other people did the same. Dorothea had been raised to believe that procrastination was the devil's work. That's why she is too embarrassed to tell her father that she has not painted her apartment like she pledged to do a year ago. It is not the case that these support group members think they are better than everyone else. They do not think well of themselves for procrastinating and therefore do not have a lot of tolerance for procrastination by others. Could the people in your life be thinking the same thing of you?

# How We Use Procrastination in Relationships

## A Way to Express Anger

Bob hated that he procrastinated. It was a bad habit he had picked up during his marriage. The marriage ended, but his procrastination didn't. He and Michelle, his ex-wife, had been very different from one another. She was beautiful and exciting. Their courtship was fun but short. They married soon after Michelle found out she was pregnant. The honeymoon didn't last any longer than the ride from Las Vegas back to Bakersfield.

Michelle moved into Bob's apartment. When they courted, she had called it their little love nest, but after they married, the place seemed inadequate. Bob had been a bachelor for a long time and lived comfortably in a two-bedroom apartment with the second bedroom serving as his "office." He had "guy stuff" all over the place. Michelle didn't like Bob's collector editions of beer bottles. Soon after the wedding she began to criticize his housekeeping abilities, his choice of décor, and his personal habits. At first Bob tried to change. He cleared out his office to make room for the baby. He threw away his favorite magazines. Those seemed like monumental sacrifices to him. But it didn't stop there. Michelle expected Bob to treat her like a "princess," which included running errands and doing chores that Bob believed would be easy for Michelle to do on her own. When he tried to say no to her, she made him feel guilty for getting her pregnant and forcing her to marry before she was ready, and Bob always gave in.

This was where his habit of procrastination started. He was angry and resented Michelle's demands. When she gave an order, he would eventually follow it, but only after putting it off as long as he could. He did not think he was being passive-aggressive. He just hated to be told what to do. He wanted to help her because he loved her, not because he was giving in. It became his habit to procrastinate until he calmed down enough to do the chore in good spirit.

The other side of the story was that Bob, although genuinely feeling bad that Michelle's life had not turned out as she had planned, was excited about being a father. He never procrastinated on any chore related to the baby. When Michelle left him and moved across the country with their daughter, Bob fell apart. His habit of procrastination grew and now affected every aspect of his life. He wanted to change. That's why he joined the support group.

## A Way to Take Control

Marta really hates being told what to do. She doesn't mind being asked. She doesn't mind working hard. She does not have a problem doing her part. But when people make demands of her or are not considerate of her time and schedule, she feels this overwhelming urge to tell them to take a flying leap.

Marta is the youngest child in her family. She has an older brother and an older sister, both of whom dumped their chores on her when she was a kid. If she didn't do what they said, they would make her life miserable. When people at work tell her what to do, she feels the same resentment. This is especially true when the person making demands on her is not higher in rank or not as smart as Marta. She wants to advance at work, so she is not in a position to speak her mind in these situations. Instead, Marta takes her time in getting things done. She is careful in how she does this. If Marta knows that the person giving her the work is supposed to do it himself and is ultimately responsible for it, Marta will intentionally delay so long that the guy is forced to take care of the task himself. This is procrastination with the purpose of teaching him a lesson.

Another way that Marta deals with people like this is to wait until the last possible minute to get things done. Marta is a fast worker, knows exactly how much time she needs, and trusts herself to meet deadlines. The person who delegated the task, however, does not know this about Marta and does not trust her, so she begins to panic as the deadline nears. Marta reassures her that she will get the job done in plenty of time, but at the same time she enjoys watching the person sweat. The reason this strategy never backfires is that Marta gets the task done and her immediate supervisor and his supervisor appreciate the speed and quality of her work.

Sometimes behavior like Marta's is referred to as passive aggression. She passively resists doing a task by procrastinating until someone else has to take action. It is aggressive in nature because the emotions behind it are negative—anger and resentment in Marta's case. The intention of the procrastination is to make others uncomfortable and to get them to do their own work, the latter being a reasonable goal in any workplace.

In Marta's case, procrastination is a way of taking control over an unpleasant situation. Her maneuver is passive but effective. So far it has not gotten her into trouble at work, but it has also not helped her achieve the goal of getting ahead. Other people who work with Marta know what she is doing. They have talked among themselves, and the word has gotten around to their superiors that Marta is not a team player. Marta thinks her team is full of idiots and resists their efforts when she thinks they are being stupid. She has self-confidence and excellent work skills, but she hates the slightest hint of being controlled. Rather than handling it in a direct way or changing jobs to get on a better team, Marta pushes back. Procrastination is one of her ways of regaining control.

Marta joined an online dating service and recently began receiving matches. Her friends had warned her about the dangers of meeting men online, but she thought it would be OK as long as she called the shots. Marta could make decisions about whom to contact, when to answer questions, when to agree to begin telephone contact, and when to meet face to face. She thought that as long as she stayed in control, things would go smoothly.

Marta was very pretty, and when men saw her photographs online, they were eager to meet her. She received many compliments and pledges of love online. She would procrastinate in responding to them just to see how long they would keep the match open before giving up on her. She was not in a hurry to settle on one man, so she took her time, giving small amounts of encouragement just to keep them in play. She got a thrill out of this and bragged to her friends that she could "string those losers along" until she was done playing with them. The downside of this strategy was that men saw through it. Some guys who would have been good choices gave up on her and closed the match. Some found other women while they were waiting on Marta's responses. Some had been in controlling relationships in the past and were sensitive to being controlled. They did not respond to her. The men who remained were those who didn't mind waiting for Marta's response or didn't catch on to her control games. Although it seemed to Marta that she was winning the online dating game, she found that she had little respect for the men who stuck it out and allowed her to control everything.

## A Way to Avoid Having to Say No

Olivia is a very sweet person, and everyone knows it. She will go out of her way to help others when she sees a genuine need. She wasn't always like that, however. Olivia used to agree to pitch in even when she knew that others could do things for themselves. Her kindness was rewarded with more and more demands. She used to have a hard time saying no to requests for her time, her cooking, and her ideas. She thought that saying no was the same as being selfish, and she thought that being selfish was sinful. She talked this over with her friends in the Procrastinators Support Group, and they set her straight.

"That's ridiculous," exclaimed Marta. "You are letting people walk all over you."

"I agree," said Dorothea. "You help a lot of people. No one could ever accuse you of being selfish with your time or talent. You are generous and giving."

"Yeah, to a fault," Bob added.

"Olivia, I bet your willingness to help makes it easier for others to say no without feeling bad about it. They know you will step in and lend a hand if they don't," Dorothea suggested. "It's OK to help when you can and say no when you can't. Try it and see how people react. I bet they will respect your assertiveness."

Olivia took their advice and found that no one reacted negatively to her newfound assertiveness. They were happy when she agreed to make their favorite dish or take the lead on a fundraiser. When she declined a request, someone else was usually willing to do it. Olivia overcame her shyness about saying no, at least some of the time.

Avoiding people can be easier than having to face the disappointed looks on their faces when you have to decline their requests. If you are sensitive to rejection, those looks can hurt even if their expressions quickly give way to acceptance or warmth. If you are accustomed to doing a lot for others and they are accustomed to asking you for help, it can be hard to make a sudden change. You feel obligated somehow, even if you are a volunteer and what you are being asked to do is not your responsibility. And others may know your weakness and use it to manipulate you into doing more. You might rely on avoiding people rather than speaking up for yourself because you think the latter will come off as confrontational. In fact, when people try to go from being pushovers to sticking up for themselves, they can overdo it and come off as aggressive. Changing Directions 15 will show you how to be assertive without going overboard and coming across as too aggressive.

Before you begin learning new ways to communicate, take a moment and read through Changing Directions 14 to find out if you are using procrastination as either a tool to make things go your way, a weapon to get back at others, or a shield to protect you from having to disappoint others.

---

↺ Changing Directions 14

## Do You Use Procrastination in Your Relationships?

Following is a summary of ways that people use procrastination to deal with relationship issues. Read through the examples and compare them to how you feel when you find yourself procrastinating rather than communicating your feelings directly with another person.

| The function of procrastination | Tool | Weapon | Shield |
|---|---|---|---|
| What procrastination expresses indirectly | Control | Anger | Fear |

| The function of procrastination | Tool | Weapon | Shield |
|---|---|---|---|
| **How you use it** | You use procrastination to control when tasks will be accomplished. | You refuse to jump when others ask you to do something. | You avoid talking to people when you think they are going to ask you to do something you would rather not do. |
| **What's behind it** | You do not like being told what to do and when and how to do it, but you do not feel comfortable saying that. | You resent the requests made by others. You do not think the person asking has the right to make demands on you. | Avoidance shields you from having to deal with people who are difficult to stand up to or say no to. |
| **Why you are afraid to speak up** | Confrontation could make matters worse. Besides, no one needs to know that you are procrastinating on purpose. | You don't want to argue. Expressing anger could get you into trouble. | You don't want the person to dislike you or think badly of you. |
| **What you tell yourself about these situations** | It's not the task that bothers me. It's who is asking and how he or she asks. | I don't want to do what they are asking, but I'm not in a position to say no. | I'm afraid to speak up for myself. I'll agree to do things just to avoid bad feelings. |

| The function of procrastination | Tool | Weapon | Shield |
|---|---|---|---|
| How it looks on the outside and feels on the inside | On the surface it may look like procrastination to others, but you know what you are doing. | On the surface you may look as if everything is fine, but on the inside you are furious. | On the surface you look like you are just too busy to talk to them, but underneath you are filled with dread. |
| The thought that goes through your mind in these situations | "You can't tell me what to do." | "You have no right to ask this of me." | "I wish you would just leave me alone." |

## A Personal Note

*I have treated couples with marital problems for many years, and what I have learned is that there are many different tools, weapons, and shields that people use to cope with stresses in relationships. Procrastination is only one of them. Anger is another commonly used vehicle. Anger can be used as a tool to make people comply with your wishes, it can be used as a weapon to attack your opponent (your spouse), and it can be used to shield you against a person's criticism, demands, or anything else you do not want to hear. Silence is another commonly used technique. Silence, also known as the silent treatment, can be used as a tool to get your partner to do what you want if you agree to start talking to him or her again once you get what you want. It can be used as a weapon if your partner hates to be ignored. Silence can also shield you from counterattack in the situation when your words might elicit a bad reaction from the other person.*

*In all of these scenarios, my goal as a marital therapist is to get the couple to use words, communicated in a respectful manner, as a tool for solving problems, expressing affection, asserting needs, and sharing intimacy. I try to encourage them to lay down their weapons and discuss issues in a rational matter. I also try to help partners become more aware of one another's sensitivities and vulnerabilities so that shields are not needed for self-protection.*

*It is always amazing to see what can be accomplished by learning to listen openly and communicate respectfully. If you have trouble doing this on your own, a marital therapist can make a great referee.*

## What to Do Instead of Procrastinating

Bob's and Marta's examples of how procrastination works in relationships show how it can be used as a way of communicating. The communication is indirect unless you tell the other person why you are stalling, avoiding, or delaying. Of course, if you were able to communicate your feelings directly, there would be no need to do it in a roundabout way. If you felt comfortable expressing your feelings directly, you could just say, "I'm upset with you and I don't want to do what you are asking right now." If Marta felt comfortable talking about how she hated being controlled by others, she could just say to men she was considering dating, "I'm not looking for a partner who wants to control everything. I like having a say in what we do." If Bob had been more comfortable, he could have told his wife how he felt about her demands, his guilt, and their marriage. If Dorothea could find the words, she could call her father and say, "Dad, I have not made time to paint the living room because I have had more important things to do. I'm concerned that you are going to make me feel bad about it when you visit." What all these statements have in common is that they are examples of assertiveness. Assertiveness is a way of directly and calmly expressing your thoughts and feelings. It is a respectful way of communicating with others. Try Changing Directions 15 and go down a different path to communicate your feelings.

↺ Changing Directions 15
## Passive–Aggressive–Assertive

To use the Goldilocks analogy, the differences among passive, aggressive, and assertive communication are that aggressive behavior is "too much" intensity in words or tone. The point being made is overshadowed by the strong emotion, so the listener hears only aggression or anger. Passivity is "too little" intensity in words or tone, so the message is not sent clearly or is lost altogether. Assertiveness is "just right." The message is sent with clear words and actions, and the tone is kept neutral so that it does not distract the listener from the point you are trying to make. If it is hard for you to be assertive, you might hold on to your words too long. When they finally come out, they may come out with much more intensity than you had planned.

Use the Who, What, Where, When, and How strategy of more assertive communication.

- **Who?** Talk directly to the person who is troubling you. Avoid complaining to others or talking behind the person's back. Marta needs to talk to those who make demands on her rather than complaining to the other staff members.

- **What?** Avoid words that will put the listener on the defensive, especially words that sound like criticism or blaming. Think about what you would want another person to say to you if you did something to upset him. Don't say more than you have to. Try not to repeat yourself. Marta could more assertively have said, "I have a lot of work to do that my supervisor already assigned me. How does this new task fit with my other priorities?"

- **Where?** Keep the discussion private. Don't humiliate the person in front of others.

- **When?** Choose a moment to communicate when you are calm and the listener has time. Speak up often. Try not to hold on to resentments.

- **How?** Keep the tone of your voice neutral. Talk about what you are feeling rather than what the other person did wrong. "I'm confused about this work you are giving me. I wasn't aware that I was supposed to do work for you."

When the Procrastinators Support Group members get together to talk, they have very little trouble being assertive with one another. Bob, who could not tell his wife how he felt about her demands, has no trouble telling Donna how he feels when she does something that gets on his nerves. Even Arthur, who is usually soft-spoken, can speak up for himself most of the time. When the issue of being assertive came up during one of their meetings, they all agreed that assertiveness is not a problem for them in the safe environment of their group or with other close friends. They all admitted, however, that when the emotional stakes seem higher, they freeze up.

## People Pleasers

Bob had been afraid to speak up for himself with his wife because he thought she would leave him. The irony is that he did not voice his feelings, and she left anyway. Dorothea wants to please her father, and she has always tried to avoid his rejection. He is not a rejecting person. In fact, he has always accepted her. She just hates his expressions of disappointment. She wants him to always be pleased with her and never disappointed. As she heard herself admit this, she felt foolish. She realized that her father does not require perfection from her. His love is unconditional. She is the one who has problems dealing with disappointed looks. Rather than scramble to make everyone approve of her at all times, she needs to learn to accept the fact that others will not find her flawless.

Trying to please other people can make you procrastinate in several different ways. It can make you avoid contact when you think someone is going to ask you do to something for her that you don't want to do, but you don't feel comfortable saying no. If you can't say no and you take on more than you can handle, you might procrastinate because you are overwhelmed and stuck. We talked about how to pace yourself in Chapter 4 on disorganization. Those strategies would work in this situation too. Another way that relationships can make you procrastinate is when you are worried that you will displease someone if you make a mistake or do something the other person won't like. In all of these cases, wanting to please others is the motivation behind agreeing to do things, and your procrastination is what happens when you freeze up with worry or dread about what they will think of you.

All of the support group members could recall times when they procrastinated in talking to someone when it would be been better to just speak their minds. Polly, for example, got a call from the church secretary asking her to once again run her church's annual choir fundraiser. She did not want to do it, but she could not find the words to say no gracefully, so she has avoided returning the call.

"I always do that," admitted Polly shyly. "I put off the call so long I have no choice but to agree to do it because it's too late to find anyone else. Then I kick myself for getting stuck with another fundraiser."

Bob admitted that he had a problem saying no to women when he felt an attraction to them. "I hate being such a stupid wimp. It didn't do me any good to let my ex-wife run all over me. I agreed to help this lady I met by repairing her kitchen cabinet. I don't really want to do it. I did not need to agree to help, and now I'm stuck. I went out with her a second time, and it didn't go very well. She keeps calling me about the cabinet. I think that's all she wants from me. I need to just tell her that I'm not interested and that I can't repair her cabinet. She can afford to hire someone to do it." The next set of Shortcuts addresses the problem of saying no. Try out these phrases or create some your own.

## ▶▶ Shortcuts for
## Saying NO

"I can't this time, but ask me next time."

"Not this time."

"Sorry, I can't help this time."

"I wish I could, but I am swamped with other things."

"I don't have enough time right now."

"I don't have enough time right now to do a good job at it."

"I'm already committed to helping with something else."

"That's not my thing. I usually help with ..."

"Can't. Sorry."

"No, I can't."

"That doesn't sound like much fun. I'll have to pass on that one."

"I'll pass, but thanks for thinking of me."

It can be difficult to start asserting yourself when you are not accustomed to doing so. It will be best if you ease into it and develop the skill over time. Following are a few suggestions for learning to become more assertive.

- Pick an easy target. Find someone who is likely to respond well to your assertiveness.

- Plan what you are going to say and practice it with a friend or in the mirror.

- Be careful not to cross over into aggression by coming on too strong.

- Try not to repeat yourself. Make your point and wait for a response.

- Don't apologize for being assertive. Just do it.

## ✑ A Personal Note

*I have been in the situation where a person has agreed to do something I have requested because he or she did not feel comfortable telling me no. I would much rather have someone tell me that she can't do something I am requesting than agree to do it and procrastinate on it because she has either no time or no desire to do it. If someone turns me down, I can find another way to solve the problem or get things done by asking another person who has more time and interest. Trying to please me by taking on more than she can handle does not do either of us any good. I have a great deal of respect for people who know their limits and can honestly assess their time availability. If I think it is important for that person to do the task, I ask her to do it even if she is limited on time or low on enthusiasm, offering to work with her to find a way to get the task done, maybe by getting her some additional assistance or relieving her of another responsibility.*

*Agreeing to do things you do not want to do or do not have time to do is not necessarily in your best interest or in the best interest of the requestor. Think about that the next time you hesitate to say no.*

# How Others Can Help You or Hurt You

Codependency is the situation where the actions of another person make it easy for your problem to continue. In the case of procrastination, if other people keep picking up the slack for you, there is no real reason for you to change. On the other hand, people who want you to stop procrastinating can help you by supporting your efforts. By sharing the two lists below you can help them understand how they might be interfering with your goal to overcome procrastination and what they can do to help you achieve lasting change. Add to the list the other ways in which people seem to help you or interfere with your plans for self-improvement. Share the list with those who are committed to helping you achieve your goals.

---

↺ Changing Directions 16

## Ways That People Can Help You or Hurt You

*Ways that people might hurt you*

- Keep doing things for you.
- Not let you know how they feel about it.
- Laugh off your procrastination.
- Lower their expectations of you.

*Ways that people can help you*

- Hold you accountable.
- Praise your efforts at change.
- Ask more of you.
- Give you a deadline.
- Check on your progress.

---

# Do You Compare Yourself to Others?

It is very common for procrastinators to assume incorrectly that other people do not procrastinate. You might even assume that others are rarely lazy. Comparing yourself to others can make you feel inferior. On the outside, however, you might try to act like you don't care or you might even be critical of nonprocrastinators, calling them names like *workaholic, compulsive,* or *anal.*

It is easy to get defensive when you feel inferior, especially when people call you out on your procrastination. You might feel compelled to justify your actions and even counterattack with statements like these:

- "I'm not lazy; I'm just taking a moment to enjoy life."
- "Don't worry about it. It will get done."
- "I'm just not as uptight as you."
- "There is more to life than work."

- "I'm not going to give myself an ulcer over this."
- "I'll do it in my own good time."

If this sounds at all like you, you are probably defensive about your procrastination. Since the best defense is a good offense, your criticism of nonprocrastinators could be just a cover for your own insecurity or guilt. Whether you are on the offense or defense, these reactions probably stem from comparing yourself to others and not feeling like you measure up.

It is not a good idea to attack others for being nonprocrastinators. It is also probably better for your relationships if you own up to your procrastination rather than pretend that it's not happening or that it is justifiable. Carla's first instinct was to get defensive, but under her strong exterior she felt ashamed and embarrassed about her behavior. Sometimes uncomfortable feelings like this can motivate you to change. It worked for Carla.

Being bothered by the idea that other people think you are a procrastinator and are disappointed in your behavior is something you can use to your advantage. The desire to prove yourself to others can be your ally in the process of change. You obviously care about your reputation. Use that to motivate yourself to change. Be the person you want others to see.

The next chapter is about all-or-nothing procrastination. This is when you either work at 100% effort or stop in your tracks and do nothing at all. This is particularly troublesome for people who are perfectionists, for those who take on more than they can handle, and for people who are "binge workers," working at full speed and then running out of steam. Even if you are not an all-or-nothing kind of person, you might find the Changing Directions exercises and Shortcuts can help you avoid procrastination.

# ⟦7⟧ All-or-Nothing Workers

**Directions:**

| | |
|---|---|
| **START:** | Acknowledge your tendency to overdo it and then shut down. |
| ➥ | Manage the feeling of being overwhelmed. |
| ➥ | Set more reasonable goals. |
| ➥ | Stop being a binge worker. |
| **END:** | Begin to pace yourself. |

There are three common types of all-or-nothing procrastinators. One group overcommits to doing things and becomes overwhelmed when there is too much to do and too little time to do it. These people tend to become immobilized when this happens. The second group of procrastinators is made up of perfectionists who will either do things perfectly or not do them at all. When they do not have the time, energy, or resources to do things the right way, they avoid the task altogether. The third group is binge workers. They go at 100 miles an hour until they run out of steam and then crash. When that happens, they stop functioning for a while and procrastinate on everything until their energy returns. This chapter will help you figure out whether you fall into any of these categories and, if so, what you can do about it.

## Avoid Feeling Overwhelmed by Overcommitment

Olivia is an overcommitter, and she knows it. She tries to do too much. She takes on big responsibilities when she could take on just a small part and share the task with others. In fact, she takes on so much sometimes that she gets overwhelmed and then completely shuts down. You might recall from the last chapter that Olivia used to be a people pleaser and would take on too much because she couldn't say no for fear of being rejected. She has managed to control that problem, but she is still a high-energy person with lots of ideas, interests, and plans, and she genuinely enjoys helping others. Olivia doesn't keep track of all the things she has going on, so she takes on more without considering how realistic it is to do so. Her enthusiasm for getting involved and her creative thinking are both good qualities, but when they lead her to assign herself more work than she can handle, it can leave her feeling overwhelmed at times. In fact, recently she has been so overwhelmed that she wants to give it all up and do nothing at all. Feeling overwhelmed is taking the pleasure out of the things that Olivia has committed herself to doing.

### ✑ *A Personal Note*

*I can identify with Olivia. I have given myself more work these days than I can realistically handle. I had a few creative ideas that led to a few new projects that have grown into big commitments. This week I am writing a research grant for myself and helping a colleague with another, finishing the edits on the last three chapters of this book, writing a final exam for my abnormal psychology class, grading 60 research papers, helping one of my students plan the last phase of her dissertation research, preparing to give two talks at international conferences, and keeping up with several large research projects that I have already started. I'm not even going to mention my family responsibilities. I have to go out of town tomorrow for a one-week "vacation," which gives me 24 more hours to finish these things before I go. It's laughable to think that I could ever get these things done. I stayed up as late as I could last night, and it is 5:00 A.M. now as I am writing to you. I feel on the verge of shutdown, only I can't give in to it because too many other people are counting on me. Everything I am working on is of my own doing—my ideas and plans. Each one seemed like a really good idea when I started. They are all coming due at the same time. None are fun anymore. I would really like to throw up my hands and say, "I can't do it," and just leave to go on vacation with no phones or e-mails to nag me. I am an overcommitter. I admit it. In my case, procrastination is not an option right now.*

Don also overcommits. He overestimates how much time he has and underestimates how long it will take to do something, and so he takes on more than he can handle, like some of the people discussed in Chapter 4. No one is forcing him. He has no trouble saying no. He just likes to take on things that he thinks he can do, should do, or would love to do, and doesn't set limits on himself until he is completely overwhelmed. Where Olivia and Don differ from people who are just disorganized or are people pleasers is that when Olivia and Don hit their limits they shut down and do nothing. Everything gets put on hold.

Although they may feel a little renewed after a lengthy period of "rest," neither Olivia nor Don can shake off the distressed feeling that comes with being overwhelmed. When going back to their activities, they do so with less enthusiasm, less energy, and less motivation. What had once seemed like a fun activity to Don or a worthwhile project to Olivia now feels like a burden. Those changes in attitude make procrastination even more likely to occur. Since both are responsible and committed people by nature, Olivia and Don will eventually see their projects through to the end, but the excitement that got them started will be replaced by relief that the projects are over. Will they overcommit the next time? You betcha!

Why? Because overcommitting is hardwired into their brains. They get a charge when they take on something new. They get excited, at least initially, when a new opportunity comes their way.

This adrenaline rush is addictive. It gives them (and me) a boost of excited energy that is positively reinforcing. When something positive, like an emotional rush, comes after a behavior, like taking on something new, it is like a reward, and rewards make us do the same thing again the next time. You could say people like Olivia and Don (and I) are overcommitment junkies.

## Kicking the Habit

You learned how to set realistic goals in Chapter 4, and in Chapter 6 you read about ways to avoid taking on things you don't really want to do just to please others. These are good tools for overcommitting caused by disorganization and difficulty saying no. If you are more like Don and Olivia (and me), though, you need to find a way out of continually burdening yourself as a result of unbridled enthusiasm, optimism, or ambition. Changing Directions 17 will help you begin to kick the habit of overcommitting.

---

↻ Changing Directions 17
### Kicking the Habit of Overcommitment

**Step 1: Stop and breathe**. A new idea or task will cause that temporary adrenaline rush that will feel like excitement. When the urge to take on something new pops into your mind, pause long enough to take a few deep breaths. Breathe in through your nose and out through your mouth, pausing for a few seconds before exhaling. Feel yourself slowing down. When the rush of adrenaline ends, you will feel calmer and more in control.

**Step 2: Stop and think it through**. Ask yourself the following questions and seriously consider the answers.

- "Why do I want to do this?"
- "Does it need to be done now?"
- "What else is on my plate right now that has higher priority?"

---

- "If I have extra time, do I really want to spend my extra time this way?"
- "Can it wait?"

**Step 3: Wait 24 hours**. Before taking on anything new, wait 24 hours. If it is still a good idea tomorrow, then you should consider doing it. If that is what you decide, use the exercises from Chapter 4 to help you organize your time. If the idea seems less important after you have had a chance to sleep on it, then drop it. Other ideas and opportunities will come your way.

## Asking for Help

Many overcommitters are also do-it-yourselfers. They aren't comfortable asking others for assistance. They would rather put something off until they have time to deal with it than admit to others that they can't do it alone. If this sounds like you, you may be thinking that there is more value in doing something yourself than in asking for help. Except for special circumstances where you get a prize for accomplishing a task on your own, there is no real advantage to being a do-it-yourselfer if it causes you to procrastinate.

Some people think that asking for help is a sign of weakness. It means that you can't handle life on your own. If this sounds like you, you have to ask yourself which is worse, showing weakness by not asking for help or showing weakness by procrastinating. It may also be helpful to know that other people don't think asking for help is a sign of weakness. In fact, most people see it as a positive trait. It gives others an opportunity to be helpful, to get closer to you, and to return the favor if you helped them, and it makes them feel good about themselves.

▶▶ Shortcuts for
## Asking for Help

If you are not accustomed to asking for help, you might need a little shove in the right direction. Following are some ideas for how you can phrase a request for assistance. Just fill in the blank with the task you have in mind.

- Do you have time to help me with my _____?

- I could use some help with _____. Do you have time to give me a hand?

- I hate to bother you, but I sure could use a hand with _____.

- Would you have any time today to help me with _____? I would be happy to return the favor.

## Perfectionistic Procrastinators

There are certain telltale signs that perfectionism is the fuel behind procrastination. One indicator is that the person is perfectionistic in several areas of his or her life. For example, he might be neat or organized or like things done a certain way. She might be a detail person who can easily spot imperfections and has a hard time ignoring them. He might have such high expectations for himself that when it is time to get something done he has to do it "right." Perfectionists procrastinate when they can't do things the way they think they should be done or the way they want them to be done. Sometimes they get stuck because they have doubts that their work will be good enough.

Sometimes perfectionists procrastinate because they think that if they start a task they can't stop until it's all done; so if they can't do it all, they won't do any of it. Sometimes that great eye for detail works against them. They feel overwhelmed by all that needs to be addressed, so they give up before they even start.

Another way that perfectionism leads to procrastination is when people get overwhelmed by the number of details required to complete a task. They think about the steps and substeps needed to get from start to finish. Polly is moving to a new house next month after living in the same place for many years. She is not moving far from her current place, but she still has to pack her belongings, clean up and paint several rooms, make repairs on her current house, and make a few changes to the new one before she moves in. When Polly looks at all that needs to be done, she can't help feeling overwhelmed by the enormity of the project. She can see what needs to be done before she can pack, while she is packing, and after she packs. There are dozens of arrangements, decisions, phone calls, and trips to the local hardware store in her future. It's more than she can handle, so she keeps putting off getting started. After Polly's mother passed away and Polly was going through a period of grief, she did not want to bathe because when she thought about bathing she thought about all the steps it would take to shampoo and condition her hair, shave her legs, thoroughly wash her body, put on lotions and deodorants, reapply her makeup, and find clothes to wear that still fit her. The thought of completing all these steps was too overwhelming, so she just didn't bathe for nearly a week.

What many perfectionists have in common is the belief that there is a right way and a wrong way to do most things. They get stuck and avoid tasks when, for whatever reason, they don't believe they can do the tasks just right. That might include not having enough time, not having the right tools, not having enough money, not getting enough cooperation from others, or not being in the right mood. "If you can't do it right, don't do it at all" was an expression Dorothea had heard throughout her childhood. Dorothea's father is a perfectionist and has little tolerance for people who are unwilling to give their all to make things turn out perfectly. He preferred to do things himself rather than settle for someone else's sloppy work. Although Dorothea resented her father's high standards while growing up, she admired his work, how he took pride in everything he did, and the products of his labor, whether it be a perfect spring garden or a perfectly painted room.

A big difference between Dorothea and her father is that she sometimes became overwhelmed by all the details involved in doing something "just right," so she would just avoid doing it. There were several things around her apartment that needed attention that she had been putting off for more than a year. For example, her living room needed a new coat of paint. The room was not very large, but it had crown moldings and baseboards that would need to be covered. The current color was dark, so she would have to prime the walls before adding the lighter shade she preferred. There were several windows with wood trim and doorjambs that would look dingy compared to the newly painted walls, so she would have to sand and prep and paint those as well. When she thought about what it would take to do it right, she decided it wasn't worth it, so she put it off. She lived alone, so no one else pushed her to do it and her father had not been to the apartment since he helped her move in. At that time, he offered to paint for her, but she declined the offer because she wanted to do it herself. She could have hired someone to paint it for her, but she didn't trust anyone but herself and her father to do it right.

Polly is also a perfectionist, and she knows it. She has high personal standards, and she worries about what others think of her. This is a dangerous combination, because it means that when she helps others she feels the need to do the job perfectly. In fact, Polly is afraid that if she does not perform up to her own personal high standards, her work will not be acceptable to others and they will think badly of her. At some level, Polly realizes that her perfectionistic standards are much higher than the standards of other people she knows, but that doesn't seem to help her. When Polly knows that she will not have the time, energy, or patience to do a task perfectly, she will avoid doing it. A good example is making a cake for a neighborhood party. Polly is a wonderful cook, and she can make most anything. Her friends look forward to potluck dinners with Polly because she always surprises the group with something new. Everyone else brings a common dish or goes to the market to purchase ready-made food. Not Polly. Polly mistakes her friends' excitement over her cooking for an expectation that she always provide the perfect dish. Sometimes Polly can't think of anything new to bring. She is afraid to bring something she has made in the past because she thinks others will be disappointed in her. Instead of looking forward to a potluck dinner with her neighborhood friends, she dreads it. She puts off her preparation until the last possible minute because she is so stressed out about the whole thing. The problem is not that Polly procrastinates when she should be cooking. The problem is that Polly's expectations for her own performance are so high that she can't fulfill them without a lot of stress. She needs help in finding the middle ground between perfect cooking and not cooking at all.

Could perfectionism be your reason for procrastinating, just like Dorothea and Polly? If it is, you might benefit from Changing Directions 18, "Finding the Middle Ground." The skill you may need is the ability to move away from an all-or-nothing approach to getting things done and toward finding a middle ground. The old view is "Do it right or don't do it at all." The new strategy is "Doing something is better than doing nothing."

---

↺ Changing Directions 18
## Find the Middle Ground

1. *What is the goal?* If you think your tendency to be perfectionistic is making you procrastinate, change directions by first defining the goal. What do you want to accomplish? Polly wants to move to her new house.
2. The second question to ask yourself is *how important it is that your goal be accomplished perfectly.* Is there any real consequence if it turns out less than perfect? Do you get any extra rewards for achieving perfection? Which will be worse, not doing it perfectly or not doing it at all? Keep in mind that just because you know how to do something perfectly does not mean you have to do it perfectly. Polly would like everything done perfectly, but the reality is that whoever buys her old home will probably redo her work. The new owner will never meet her, so it doesn't matter what he or she thinks of Polly's cleaning job. The only reward for Polly is that she feels satisfaction when she can do something perfectly. Right now she only feels dread as the time left before the move is passing quickly.
3. Find the middle. *If at one extreme is procrastination and on the other extreme is perfection, what is in the middle?* The middle

---

might include doing part of a task instead of procrastinating, doing a little at a time, letting someone else do it for you, or doing it all but lowering the standard a bit. Polly decided to put her perfectionistic energy into her new home rather than into cleaning her old home. In fact, since she will move into her new house before selling her old one, she will work on the new one first. If she runs out of time or energy, she will ask someone to help her clean up the old house.

4. Tell yourself that *it is better to do something than to do nothing* and take a step toward your goal. Polly agrees that doing nothing is a problem and taking any step in the right direction is better than staying stuck. She decided that her first step will be to plan where she will put her furniture in her new house. She is also going to stop herself from planning every single detail of the move and making herself feel overwhelmed. She will take one step at a time, and the first step is to write down her ideas for transferring her furniture from the old house to the new one.

To get started on finding a middle ground, Dorothea defined her goal, which was pretty simple: to paint the living room a lighter color. When she then looked at how important perfection in painting it would be, she had to admit that there was no reward for painting her living room perfectly. The only possible consequence was that if her father visited he would notice the imperfections. He probably would not say anything about it, but Dorothea would know that he had noticed. When she asked herself if it would be worse for her father to notice her imperfections or for him to see that she had never painted the room at all, she thought the latter would be a bigger problem. On second thought, what Dad thought was not really the issue; she was tired of looking at the ugly wall color and wanted to change it. She would rather paint it less than perfectly than continue to look at it the way it was. As a middle ground, Dorothea chose to give up the goal of painting everything perfectly, like her father would do, and just cover up the old color of her walls with a primer paint. Primers do not have to be done perfectly. Their function is to cover old ugly paint, and that is all that Dorothea wanted. If she has time left, she will go ahead and paint over the primer.

## Binge Workers

Terry feels like she is always behind schedule. She has little kids, works at a local elementary school, and keeps up with household and family responsibilities. Her husband travels a lot for his job. Terry is a "binge worker." She has a hard time getting started with chores, but once she starts she can't stop. Terry pushes herself to the point of exhaustion and then collapses. Once she has hit her limit, she can't do any more for hours or sometimes for days at a time. While she is resting up to regain her strength, a new mountain of chores is growing. Terry doesn't have the energy to take them on, so she lets them accumulate until she has the strength and then binge works again.

In addition to overcommitting, Don and Olivia also take an all-or-nothing approach to work. They either go full speed ahead or stop dead in their tracks. When the latter happens, they go fishing or park themselves in front of the television and do nothing. They ignore phone calls, e-mails, text messages, faxes, and knocks at the door. Don sits on the couch in his underwear and doesn't even want to take a shower. Olivia stays in bed all day. Eventually, they both find a way out of the deep dark well they have fallen into and begin again to take on their tasks.

The intervention for binge working is to pace yourself, rest when you need it, and set smaller goals for yourself. If you do not become overwhelmed with fatigue, you will not shut down. Try not to be like Terry, who thinks she doesn't deserve a break unless she is caught up on everything. Give yourself permission to do your chores at a reasonable pace. Take a breather now and look over the following Shortcuts for binge workers.

⏭ Shortcuts for
## Binge Workers

1. Set an alarm every few hours as a reminder to have lunch, take bathroom breaks, and drink water.

2. Breathe. Take a deep breath after each step you accomplish.

3. Stretch periodically. Work out the kinks before you continue to work.

4. Check the time occasionally to monitor your working hours.

5. From time to time, stop working and admire your progress.

6. Monitor your energy level.

7. Stop working before you completely run out of energy.

Go back to the time management exercises in Chapter 4 to learn how not to overestimate what you can do and underestimate the amount of time you have to do it. Plan your activity around your energy level. If you know you have enough steam to last for three hours, then plan only three hours of work. If you know you are a morning person and not an evening person, plan to do more when you first wake up. Keep in mind that you will probably begin by overestimating how much energy you have. You will need to learn your limits by comparing your estimated time against your reality. Pay attention to the onset of fatigue. That will be your clue that you have run out of steam. The signs of fatigue can be physical, like low energy, muscle aches, hunger, thirst, or blurred vision. They can be mental, such as loss of concentration, or emotional, such as irritability, anxiety, or agitation. You might start to make mistakes, drop your tools, or lose coordination. You don't have to wait for all of these signs to appear to know you have had enough.

## *Know Your Limits*

Procrastination can vary with your energy level; less energy means more procrastination. Everyone has natural fluctuations in energy levels throughout the day and over time. That means procrastination will also fluctuate over time. Some people procrastinate more in the morning than in the afternoon, or vice versa, depending on when they have the most energy. You can plan your work around naturally occurring surges and drops in your energy during the day or during certain days of the week. Pick the time when you are at your best and take action during those times.

Arthur, for example, does his best work at night. He is not a morning person. Nonetheless, he occasionally makes plans to get up early to do chores. He sets the alarm to get up an hour early, hits the snooze button a few times, and eventually makes himself get out of bed and shower. However, this slow process takes up much of the extra time he thought he would have to work. With the time he has left before he has to go to work, he tries to get a few things done, but he is clearly not at his best. The problem is not that Arthur can't get out of bed earlier. The problem is that his energy is too low in the morning to do chores, especially those that take a lot of mental energy. It would be better for Arthur if he planned to do his extra chores in the evening or during his lunch hour, when he is alert and ready to work.

Pay attention to your energy level. Even if it seems logical to get up a little earlier to catch up on things you have avoided, it may not be the most efficient thing to do. Don't set yourself up for failure trying to fix your procrastination by doing your extra chores when you know you will not be at your best. Know your limits and make your plans for when you are most likely to be successful.

▶▶ Shortcuts for
## Fluctuating Hormones

For women, energy can fluctuate with hormonal changes during the menstrual cycle. It is not unusual for mood and energy to be lower than usual premenstrually and once your period begins. Some women experience similar changes at the time of ovulation, although more briefly.

If mood and energy are low, there is a good chance motivation will be low and you will be more likely to procrastinate. Setting smaller goals to match your energy level is one way to cope during these times. Another is to make sure you get enough sleep and keep a normal meal schedule. Keep in mind that just because your hormones may make it a little harder to overcome procrastination does not mean that you can't do anything about it.

Consider keeping a diary for a few months about your hormone fluctuations and how they affect your energy, motivation, and procrastination. Find out if there is a pattern to it for you. Diaries can take many forms, from the traditional booklike diary to a simple rating on your monthly calendar such as 10 for high energy to 0 for no energy. You won't believe that hormones have anything to do with it until you see it for yourself. Once you are convinced by your own diary entries, you can begin to plan ahead for the next cycle. Give it a try.

## ✄ A Personal Note

*Today I was reminded of the exhilaration that comes with being caught up on tasks. I have been behind for some time on a number of important tasks—some for work, some for family, some personal, some for friends. While I have not missed any real deadlines like the kind for filing tax returns or paying rent, I have missed my own personal deadlines a dozen times. I have made the same promise to myself, that I will get something done by the end of the week, more times than I would like to admit.*

*Having said this, I promised myself I would get caught up on a number of nagging tasks by the time the new semester started. It did not happen the way I had planned. It seems like every time I make a plan to catch up, something else interferes with my plans. I get sick or someone in my family needs help or a new opportunity with a short deadline comes my way. Every time I turned around there was something new to sabotage my efforts to be productive. It was really stressing me out. Finally, the last week before classes started back up, I got a break.*

*Over the course of a week, I took care of all the nagging little tasks that had been on my mind and the big difficult tasks that needed to be done. I had imagined letting people down on the things that had to do with others, but all were pleased to hear from me, and none were inconvenienced by my tardiness. That was a relief. I mailed out all the work-related things that needed to be finished, and that was an even bigger relief. In going through the piles of paper on my desk, I realized there were several things I had already taken care of but forgotten to remove from the pile. They just needed to be filed or shredded or thrown away. When I looked up from my work at the end of the last day of playing catch-up, I realized that I could actually see the bottom of my in-box. It's black shiny plastic that has not been marked or faded like the rest of the box because it has not seen the light of day in months. Wow, what a sense of accomplishment.*

*I wanted to hold on to that feeling in hopes that it would motivate me to stay ahead, not procrastinate, not get behind. I put on my running shoes and went out for a celebratory run. I memorized the feelings of relief and satisfaction. I patted myself on the back. I felt like Rocky running to the top of the Philadelphia Museum of Art's front steps. I raised my hands in triumph and took a mental picture of myself. I like that feeling. I want that feeling all the time.*

*After bragging to my husband and sons and friends and the lady at the checkout stand at my local grocery store (she was especially impressed and envied my accomplishment), something a little discouraging occurred to me. This feeling of success and joy and relief came only after I had dug myself out of a pit of backlogged work. If I stayed caught up, I would feel good about it, but not exhilarated.*

*So the feeling I memorized is something I would never feel again unless I allowed another pile of work and guilt to accumulate. What a thought! Could it be that I intentionally get behind just so I can feel the joy of catching up? Surely that can't be what is happening to me, but it is definitely worth considering. Would I be willing to give up those Rockyesque moments by staying on top of things? That's a good question.*

## Find a Balance between Work and Play

The word *balance* is misleading. Balance assumes some type of equality or equal weighting of our work responsibilities and pleasurable activities. For adults, most of our time is taken up tending to responsibilities at work, at home, and with our families. It is not physically possible to balance those hours with recreation, pleasure, or relaxation. We have a limited number of waking hours in our day.

Procrastination can be a way that we try to regain "balance" by putting aside chores, tasks, responsibilities, and obligations and taking time to relax. In fact, for some people, procrastination may be the only way to find time to relax. A better way to look at it is that those who have a lot to do will have no time left in their schedules to relax unless they intentionally stop working for a while. This is not quite the same as procrastination. It is more like making time to relax and rest.

Those who are not overburdened with responsibilities still need to take time to enjoy life. They need to find "balance" in a different way. True procrastinators stop being productive when their lives are full of obligations and not enough pleasant experiences. They need a certain amount of play time to make their work time seem less burdensome. If this sounds like you, the challenge is to have enough pleasurable time without overdoing it. You run the risk of fooling yourself into believing you need more time off than is necessary. Go back to Chapter 4 and read the section on fooling yourself to help you find the balance between too little and too much pleasure.

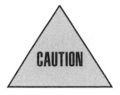

## A Word of Warning

There is a difference between having skills and using them. You might have read through this chapter and realized you already possess the practical skills described. You just may not be using them. Knowing how to do something does not necessarily translate directly into behavior change. Make it your goal to begin to put your knowledge and skills into action. Keep it simple. Just try to procrastinate less next week than you have this week.

The next chapter addresses a question that is often on the minds of procrastinators: "Am I just lazy?" It is a good question. If you have made it this far through the book and have not found a reason for your procrastination, perhaps it is just a preference for recreation, pleasure seeking, or rest. While there is nothing wrong with these preferences in moderation, you probably started reading this book and stuck with it this far because you think you are overdoing it. Read on and find out if laziness and pleasure seeking are behind your procrastination.

# 8  Pleasure Seekers

**Directions:** 

> **START:** Figure out whether laziness is your problem.
>
> ➡ Understand the social consequences of procrastination.
>
> ➡ Find out how you might have been trained to let others do your work.
>
> ➡ Learn to transition from pleasure seeking to taking action.
>
> **END:** Set realistic goals for pleasure seeking and work.

## "Maybe I'm Just Lazy"

The members of the Procrastinators Support Group Chapter 121 talk a lot about laziness. In fact, most of them assumed that their procrastination was simply a sign of laziness and a preference for pleasure over work. As they have struggled with the various causes of procrastination, they have come to realize that there are times when laziness is what makes them procrastinate especially when they don't feel like doing the work at hand. To try to understand themselves better, they made an effort to learn to distinguish laziness and pleasure seeking from the other types of procrastination. Here are some of the examples of pleasure-seeking procrastination that they came up with:

- When you could easily make yourself something healthy to eat because you have the food, the time, and the energy, but you eat a big bag of chips instead.

- When you would have to walk only three feet to put your clothes in a hamper, but instead you drop them on the floor.
- When you don't mind doing a chore at home and you have the time to do it, but you watch TV instead.
- When you have had enough sleep and you are looking forward to starting your day, but you want 5 more minutes of sleep anyway.
- When it would take less time to walk somewhere than to drive your car and find a parking space and you drive anyway.
- When you drink out of the milk carton instead of pouring the milk into a glass, even though a glass is easily accessible.
- When you choose to lie down because it takes less energy than sitting.
- When you leave an empty box of cereal on the counter next to the trash can.
- When you watch something stupid on TV because that takes less energy than getting up to find the remote.
- When you drive your car down the driveway to get the mail, even when it is close enough to walk.
- When you delay doing a chore because you know your mother will get disgusted and eventually do it for you.
- When you wear your roommate's clothes that are not exactly your size because you don't want to do laundry.

If you do any of these things or something similar, your reason for procrastinating might be pleasure seeking. This doesn't mean that the other reasons for procrastinating do not apply to you. We procrastinate for different reasons at different times and in different situations. Maybe you hesitate to take action for a very good reason when the task is stressful or challenging, and maybe sometimes you just don't want to move. It is OK to admit that. There is nothing wrong with preferring pleasure over work. It is good to take the easier path, to allow yourself time to relax and enjoy the moment, and to slow down from time to time. This chapter includes tips for dealing with the kind of procrastination that simply comes from laziness and pleasure seeking.

## ✍ *A Personal Note*

*Pleasure seeking is usually a good thing. I enjoy my work, but given the choice, I would rather play. That's if I could play without having to think about work. That is what vacations are for. Although I always have enough work to keep me busy year round, I have discovered that I am a happier person if I take time to play. Pleasurable activities revitalize me. They add joy to a life full of work and challenges. When I return from vacation, I have more energy to take on whatever faces me. This is my justification for taking time off to relax or goof off.*

*In reality, there is always work to do. When I come home from work, I am always faced with household chores. When my children were younger and living at home, there were always kid-related things to do. I get lots of phone calls after work, and some are about tasks I need to complete. I could fill every hour of my day with work and still not be caught up. When I was growing up, my mother would always tell me to get my work done before I played. That was easier to do when I was nine years old. Now that I'm an adult, her rule doesn't work for me because if I tried to follow it I would never have time to play.*

*I put off chores to have fun. This is one form of procrastination. Usually I can set limits on it and get back to work. However, if it has been a particularly difficult week at work and I have put in lots of late hours, I have much more trouble motivating myself to stop playing and get back to my chores.*

## "Mom Will Do It"

In the first chapter, I told you that one of the reasons we procrastinate is because we can. We get away with it. One of the reasons we get away with it is that other people sometimes get impatient with us and do the task for us. These individuals might be mothers, partners, spouses, roommates, girlfriends, or coworkers. They do things for us because they reach a limit and can no longer tolerate waiting for us to take action. We could be cold about it and say, "That's their problem, not mine," but that is just a thing we say to hide shame or guilt.

In psychological terms we call this process *positive reinforcement* for procrastination. You procrastinate and in turn get rewarded by someone who will do the work for you. It seems like a win-win situation because these other people get the task done, which makes them feel better, and you get out of having to do it, which makes you feel better. The way positive reinforcement works, however, is that once you are rewarded for your procrastination you are more likely to do it again. A common example is a mother who tells her child to pick up his toys. The child says, "I'll do it in a minute." The mother reminds him about the toys a few more times and then gives in and picks them up and puts them away. The child is scolded about it but replies with "I was just about to do it." This, of course, is not completely honest, but the child thinks it relieves him of blame for not picking up the toys. His mother has inadvertently rewarded the child for procrastinating by doing the work for him. That means he will likely do it again next time.

That boy will then grow up to be a man with a live-in girlfriend or wife. He will probably pick a woman who is like his mother, tidy and organized in her environment, because he likes a neat home. She will ask him to pick up his socks, take out the trash, or put away his shoes, and he will respond with "I'll do it in a minute. I'm in the middle of something right now." He knows, at least subconsciously, that if he does not move fast enough, she will do it for him. He is right. She picks up his dirty socks, stinky underwear, or smelly shoes and puts them where they belong. She tells herself that she should not have to do this and that his mother should have taught him how to pick up after himself (they always blame the mother). Getting yucky things off the floor makes her feel better, and not having to do the chore makes him feel better. It is another win-win situation. If this sounds like you, it's not because your girlfriend thinks she is your mother. It would also not be fair to say it is not your fault and that you are just a victim of poor parenting.

You might be wondering why you would need to change a win-win situation. The reason is that people don't feel very good about doing chores for you and don't feel good about you. With the exception of your mother, others who have to pick up the slack for you will begin to resent you. They feel you are taking advantage of them. In all honesty, you probably *are* taking advantage of them.

If you are otherwise a likable person, your friends probably learn to accept your laziness and procrastination. For example, procrastinators are often late for appointments. Other people anticipate this tardiness and schedule around it. They might tell you to arrive at 9:00 for an event that doesn't actually start until 10:00. Even when people are good-natured about it, your tardiness, inertia, or procrastination has a negative effect. Other people begin to view you as untrustworthy or irresponsible. They don't take you as seriously as you would like. You exhaust their tolerance and patience on small, stupid things you could very well do for yourself. After a while they begin to feel resentful, they lose their patience, and overreact when they reach their limit.

There is a price to pay for all forms of procrastination. When your pleasure seeking negatively impacts others, the price is a change in their feelings toward you. Perhaps keeping the respect of others is worth the effort of picking up your own socks or showing up on time so others can count on you.

Evelyn falls into this category of procrastination. She has a wonderful mother who has taken very good care of Evelyn, helped her, nurtured her, and fussed over her. There have been many times when Evelyn knew she could do things for herself, like prepare her own lunch, but she let her mother do it for her. She justified it by telling herself that her mom enjoyed taking care of her, but Evelyn knew in her heart of hearts that she was just lazy and she liked it when her mother did things for her.

When Evelyn's mom took a second job to help pay for Evelyn's college tuition, Evelyn felt bad about it. She saw the fatigue on her mother's face but let her continue to cook and clean for Evelyn whenever she was at home on breaks from school. Her mom never seemed to resent the extra work, but Evelyn knew she was taking advantage of the situation and that her siblings and father thought less of her for it. She needed to stop being lazy and take more responsibility before her mother began to resent her too.

## ৯ *A Personal Note*

*In some ways, I have been very lucky. My husband's parents made him take a lot of responsibility for himself and for his brothers at a very young age. When we met in high school, he did not expect me to serve him. I liked this because I had dated other boys who expected me to take care of them as their mothers had. My mother and father, however, ruined things for me by spoiling my husband. My husband loved the way my mother fussed over him, and he showed his gratitude regularly. My father would get after me if I seemed to be neglecting my husband's needs because he believed that it was the woman's place to serve her husband. My mother had spoiled my father too. Being young and still obedient to my parents, I began to do things for my husband that he could clearly do for himself. He loved it, and my parents were proud that I was becoming a good wife. My husband wrongly assumed that I enjoyed doing things for him even when he could do them himself, so he continued to make requests. When we began to have children and I started to go to graduate school, I could no longer keep up with my "wifely responsibilities." I tried to explain this to my husband, but he did not quite get it. He continued to expect me to do things that he could easily do. If I asked that he take care of something himself, he would procrastinate until the problem hit a crisis level and I had to take care of it. This was when his behavior crossed the line from enjoying the loving care of a giving wife to being just plain lazy. Even though I tried to make it clear that he needed to go back to fending for himself while I took care of our home, the kids, and my education and career, he held on to the fantasy that, like my mother, I enjoyed spoiling him.*

*After years of disagreement, compromise, and adjustment, we* have found a balance between serving each other and fending for ourselves. Because he does not demand it all the time, I do things for him because I enjoy it. He returns the favor by doing things for me just because it makes him feel good. This balance works most of the time. The only time we slip into old patterns is when my godmother visits and spoils my husband just as my mom used to do. He loves her very much and loves how she cooks for him and fusses over him. When she leaves, it takes me a few weeks to train him back into balance.

## Making the Transition from Laziness to Taking Action

Procrastination due to laziness gives us internal rewards. We feel pleasure when we are doing something fun instead of having to do something unpleasant. Playing computer games is an example. Winning a hand of solitaire, especially the more challenging games, is rewarding. If we are playing the game instead of doing homework or cleaning the kitchen or working on our taxes, it makes the win just that much sweeter. Unfortunately, while we sit in front of the computer or the television or a good book, thoughts of what we need to be doing can creep back into our minds and spoil the fun. That makes our procrastination not so rewarding anymore. When something stops giving us pleasure and stops being rewarding, it is time to stop doing it. The next exercise provides some clues to help you know when it is time to transition from pleasure seeking to work.

---

↺ Changing Directions 19

### Learn When to Stop Pleasure Seeking

You can allow some pleasure seeking, but set limits on how much time you spend doing it. Here are some examples of how to know when you have hit your limit on pleasure seeking and it is time to get back to work. Use these cues to know when it is time to change gears.

---

## Feel the downshift:

- It's time to shift gears when the activity you are doing stops being enjoyable and starts to feel repetitive or boring or you become aware that you are doing it just to avoid work. Break up the boredom by replacing it with the feeling of accomplishment. Take action.

- When you are running out of time to get a task done and you feel the pressure starting to make you tense, you should relieve the stress by switching your focus to accomplishing your goals.

- If your mind starts to fill with worries, rumination, or preoccupation with chores while you are trying to have fun, you have shifted out of the pleasure zone of procrastination. That means it is time to stop playing. Relieve your stress by doing something productive. Doing something usually feels better than doing nothing in these situations.

## Watch for the signs:

- The impatience or repeated nagging of others can be a sign that it is probably time to stop procrastinating and get moving. Turn off their noise by addressing their concerns. It will make you feel better too.

- When watching a little TV turns into a sitcom marathon of shows you have already seen, perhaps more than once, this is a sign that you are not just enjoying TV, you are procrastinating on other things. When the next episode is over, it is time to turn it off.

- If you smell bad because you have delayed showering or you are still wearing yesterday's clothes, you have procrastinated a little too long. Time to take a bath. Feeling refreshed will motivate you.

- When you start to feel bad about yourself or call yourself lazy, you may be signaling to yourself that it is time to change directions. Do something that will leave you feeling successful, relieved, or less burdened.

*Look ahead for roadblocks:*

- If not taking action is going to eventually cause you trouble, your procrastination has become self-defeating. Rather than give yourself another reason to feel bad, take at least one step toward your goal. If that feels good, take another step. It will pay off.

- When you know that playing instead of working is going to put you behind and add to tomorrow's workload or lead to a stressful situation where you feel pressed for time, you should set limits on your procrastination. Rather than living for the moment, look at the big picture and plan ahead.

Arthur really enjoys *Law and Order* reruns. His favorite is the *Criminal Intent* series, but he also likes the others. He uses his DVR to identify and then record all of the *Law and Order* shows whenever they are aired, which is often when he is at work. If he is tied up with work or with group meetings or other activities in the evenings, he may not be able to watch the shows until the weekend. When that happens, he sometimes gets hooked on them and will watch them all in one sitting. Hours can pass while he sits on the sofa in his boxers, unbathed and unshaven, relaxing in the peace of his quiet home. Unfortunately, Arthur usually has a lot to do on the weekends, like housekeeping, home repairs, or work left over from his job. He knows these things need to get done, and he has a hard time not thinking about them while he is watching television. By about the third episode of *Law and Order*, Arthur can feel the downshift in his mood. His guilty conscience for being lazy instead of working starts to ruin his pleasure. He can ignore it temporarily, but by the time he gets through a week's worth of reruns, he often feels pretty lousy (and he smells bad too).

When the Procrastinators Support Group talked about the difference between laziness and procrastination, it became clearer to Arthur that he had been feeling the shift from pleasure to discomfort when he watched TV, but he had been ignoring the signs. At some level he was aware that his enjoyment began to decline after a while as his anxiety began to increase. When that happened, he would pause the DVR and get something to drink or find a snack. That broke the tension temporarily and allowed him to go back to his reruns. Now that the group was talking about it, Arthur decided to change this pattern. It seemed dumb to him to watch reruns so much that they became unenjoyable. That defeated the whole purpose of recording the shows when he was at work. He just needed to find a way to disengage from the TV and switch his focus to things that would make him feel better about himself, such as changing burned-out light bulbs in his house or washing the dishes.

## ✎ *A Personal Note*

*I am writing this on a beautiful day in the late winter when the weather is finally good enough to go outside and do some yard work. I can see through the window all that needs to be done. I also know there is laundry to do and there are a few things from work I should probably finish, but it is the weekend and I am enjoying sitting here in front of my computer. Before I opened this file to begin writing, I was playing a new version of solitaire that I downloaded yesterday. After a few games, I started thinking that I should probably get a few things done this morning. The longer I played, the longer the list got and the more pressure I was feeling to go do some work. The solitaire game stopped being fun. I continued to play for a few more hands, thinking I would shake off the feeling of guilt for being lazy instead of working, but it didn't go away. Not yet feeling motivated to do chores, I compromised and opened my word-processing program to work on this book. Technically, I am working while I write to you, but I enjoy writing, so it never really feels like work (unless my editor is nagging me).*

Sometimes to go from procrastinating to working you need a transition step. Most people who procrastinate have a hard time bouncing up from the couch and going straight to a difficult or unpleasant task. Smaller steps can help you ease into it. Once you are moving, it is easier to keep moving. The hardest part is getting started. Changing Directions 20 will help you transition from pleasure seeking to more productive activities.

---

↺ Changing Directions 20

## Making the Transition from Pleasure Seeking to Work

**Step 1: Gain self-awareness.** If you have made it this far in the book, you have obviously begun to consider your procrastination a problem worth addressing. That is an important first step. If you think you need to make some change in your behavior, then you have accomplished Step 1.

**Step 2: Notice when you are procrastinating and admit it to yourself.** You can use the clues from Changing Directions 19 to help catch the pleasure-seeking kind of procrastination when it is happening.

**Step 3: Identify what you should be doing instead of pleasure seeking.** If there are many tasks that need to be completed, focus on the one that you are most likely to do. It doesn't have to be the most important task. It just needs to be something you can envision yourself doing. Hold that picture in your mind for a few moments and find a reason it would be good for you to transition from having fun to doing that task.

**Step 4: Take a step away from pleasure seeking.** Do a small task or chore that would be quick or easy to complete. Let's say you are procrastinating on chores such as cleaning the kitchen. Start by emptying the trash can, turning on the dryer to fluff the clothes you left there overnight, or putting away some things that you left lying around the house. These chores are small enough not to be painful, and they serve the purpose of getting you moving.

---

> **Step 5: Pat yourself on the back**. Acknowledge that you were able to move yourself from pleasure seeking to work. Noting your successes in overcoming procrastination will reinforce your efforts and give you a sense of accomplishment.

Arthur decided to try breaking away from his *Law and Order* marathon by trying the exercise in Changing Directions 20. He was aware that he started to feel uncomfortable after watching a few episodes, especially if he had not yet bathed and dressed for the day. He knew that feeling uncomfortable is what would make him go to the kitchen for food or something to drink. When he was getting his snack, he usually noticed the dishes in the sink or the overflowing trash can but told himself he would get to it after the next episode. Arthur had to admit that this was his pattern just about every Saturday. He wanted to change. Arthur's plan was to try Step 2 and catch his procrastination right when it was happening. In fact, the next weekend when he started to watch TV, he realized after the first episode that he was already feeling a little uncomfortable. He was so excited that he caught the feeling right when it happened that he turned off the TV right away. Arthur remembered that Step 3 was to pick a task or chore that needed to be done, so he picked cleaning his bedroom. He needed to straighten things up, change the sheets on his bed, vacuum the carpet, dust the furniture, and put away his shoes. None of these were fun to do, but he decided to try Step 4 by putting his shoes away and then pulling the sheets off the bed. After doing that, Arthur turned *Law and Order* back on and watched another episode. When it was over, he went to the laundry room to find some clean sheets for his bed. He took the vacuum cleaner out of the closet and found some furniture polish and a cloth. He was just about to go watch more television when he realized that it would take all day to clean his room at this pace. Instead, he finished the task, took a shower, made himself some lunch, and then sat in his favorite chair to enjoy the rest of his taped shows. He noted that he felt good about what he had done and also admitted that it wasn't that difficult to do. He just had a tendency to make chores seem more unpleasant in his mind.

## "I Don't Care"

Apathy is an emotion that commonly causes procrastination. Do you procrastinate because you really don't care? Or do you procrastinate for other reasons and eventually get so far behind that you stop caring? Bob started procrastinating as a way of getting back at his demanding wife. He fell farther and farther behind. She left him, and he just stopped caring. His apathy may have been a result of sadness or grief, but if you asked Bob, he would just say he didn't care.

People who procrastinate on chores are sometimes criticized by others for their slovenliness. They are called names like *slob* or *lazy bum*. These people procrastinate in doing laundry, washing their cars, mowing their lawns, or getting a haircut. If you ask them about it, they might say they don't care. They ignore the criticism, and they get around to doing these chores when it is convenient for them.

There is more to not caring than meets the eye. On the surface it may look like normal pleasure seeking, but if this attitude carries over to many areas of life, it may be a sign of a more significant problem. Apathy and procrastination can be a sign of depression or distress. If it is just pleasure seeking, you will experience positive emotions while procrastinating. If it is part of a bigger problem like depression, apathy will be accompanied by low energy, low motivation, sleeping problems, changes in appetite, poor concentration, a low mood, and sometimes feelings of hopelessness, helplessness, or worthlessness. If you experience these symptoms, talk with your doctor. If you want to know more about the signs of depression, go online to *www.dbsalliance.org*. The Depression and Bipolar Support Alliance has information about several types of depression and ideas for where to go for help.

Sometimes Freddie thinks he is depressed. He really has no

excuse for being lazy as often as he is. His pleasure seeking goes way beyond what most people do. His motivation has been low since his teenage years. He has often wondered if there was something more seriously wrong with him. He looked online for the symptoms of depression, and he thinks he may have something called *dysthymic disorder*. As soon as his mom feels better, Freddie is going to make an appointment with his doctor and check it out.

## Commitment to Change

At the end of the first chapter the roadmap for change was described. As you read through this book, you were evaluating yourself, thinking of opportunities for improvement, and learning new skills that would help you gain control over your tendency to procrastinate. Each chapter helped you identify the reasons behind your procrastination and what you could do to address those problems more directly. In this chapter you learned to distinguish laziness from those other types of procrastination. You have probably figured out that you procrastinate for many different reasons, depending on the situation. As we near the end of this book, it's time to begin putting the pieces together.

Changing your pattern of procrastination is like breaking any bad habit. You have to find a reason to change, set a goal, and work slowly toward self-improvement. This is true regardless of what kind of procrastinator you might be. The next Changing Directions exercise (no. 21) will walk you through the steps of making big changes in your tendency to procrastinate. Its focus is on behavior change. If you procrastinate for reasons other than laziness, you should work through the exercises for your type of procrastination in addition to doing the following exercise. The Changing Directions and Shortcut interventions that were described within the other chapters will help you overcome the specific problems that underlie your tendency to procrastinate. Changing Directions 21 picks up where those exercises leave off. It assumes you have taken time to address your unique problem with procrastination.

---

↻ Changing Directions 21

## How to Break the Habit of Procrastination

**Step 1: Find a reason to change**. There is a reason you decided to buy this book and take on the problem of procrastination. You (or the person who gave you this book) realize how procrastination is negatively affecting your life. From what you have learned so far about procrastination, identify the most compelling or powerful reason for change. Say your reason out loud to yourself and write it on the line below.

My reason for changing my habit of procrastinating is: _____

_____

---

Evelyn's reason to change is so her mother will stop feeling the need to take care of her and will not begin to resent her.

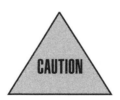

Do not commit yourself to change because you think it will please another person or get someone off your back. Your plan for permanent change will succeed only if you have a personal reason for wanting to control your procrastination. Be honest with yourself. If you are not ready to change or you are not convinced that you need to change, you are better off waiting until you think it would be helpful to you.

Evelyn understands that her mother has wanted her to be responsible all her life. It will please her mother if she makes changes now. But it will also please Evelyn if she can be a "better person" and not such a pleasure seeker. She sees this as an opportunity for another win-win situation. Her mother will be happy. She will be happy that her mother is happy, and she will be proud of herself.

**Step 2: Pick a target**. You can't stop being a procrastinator all at once. You have to do it in stages, by choosing one thing at a time to change. For example, you might want to stop procrastinating on filing your taxes this year, or you might want to stop procrastinating on your homework.

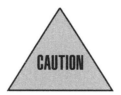

Don't start with the hardest task first. Pick something that might be easy to fix, such as something that you procrastinate on only half of the time.

**Step 3: Set a realistic goal**. It is difficult to change from being a daily procrastinator to someone who never delays on things. In fact, since some procrastination is perfectly normal, your goal should be to reduce your procrastination rather than eliminate it altogether.

Aim for improvement over short time periods, such as procrastinating less on your homework this week than you did last week. Don't try to quit cold turkey. If you fail in the first week, you will very likely give up your efforts to change.

Arthur is going to make his goal to keep his home in better condition. He avoids having people over because it is a mess. If he watched less TV and cleaned up at home, he could have the support group members over for dinner and not feel embarrassed by his surroundings. The way he handled his *Law and Order* watching and doing chores seemed like a good routine. If he did a little bit each weekend, he could have his home looking good in about a month. That would make him feel good and would allow him to have friends over, which would make him feel good too.

> **Step 4: Take a step in the right direction.** If you have gotten this far in the book, you have already made progress toward improvement. You have made a decision to try to better understand your problem. Keep going by taking another step toward freedom from procrastination.

The right direction for you might be to be less of a pleasure seeker, or it might be to address your unique reason for procrastinating. Make a commitment to yourself to work through the exercises in this book, to reread chapters, or to talk it over with a friend. It took you a while to become a procrastinator, and it will take a little while to learn to procrastinate less. Set your goal at making tomorrow better than today or next week better than this week. Before you know it, you will have control over when you choose to procrastinate and when you choose not to.

## Why Change When This Is Working for You?

The downside of changing is that you will have to greatly reduce your pleasure-seeking ways and take care of things on your own. This is difficult to do because, given the choice, many people would rather be served than have to exert energy to take care of themselves. You have to be pretty motivated to give up some of the goodies that go with procrastination.

Throughout the chapters of this book, beginning in Chapter 2, the exercises have asked you to identify reasons to change—to stop procrastinating. You have had time to consider the factors that might be making you procrastinate. You have read about the advantages and the disadvantages of using procrastination as your way of coping with life.

You know that procrastination is an easier path to go down than the path to change. And you know that you can get away with procrastination without any serious consequences a great deal of the time. If you still want to change your ways, you must have some pretty good reasons to challenge yourself now. In Changing Directions 22, it is time to summarize what you have figured out so far about yourself and your procrastination. Take your time, think it through, and jot down the most compelling and important reasons you have for making changes in your tendency to procrastinate.

---

↺ Changing Directions 22
## Reasons to Change

Now that you are more aware of why you procrastinate and what you need to change, take some time to review your motivation for change. Fill in the blanks to begin to strengthen your commitment to controlling procrastination.

1. Reasons it would be better for my relationships if I stopped procrastinating:

   _____

   _____

2. Ways that my self-image would change if I stopped procrastinating:

   _____

   _____

3. How my life would improve if I procrastinated less:

   _____

   _____

4. What others would think of me if I procrastinated less:

   _____

   _____

---

In the next and final chapter, you will learn how to make lasting changes in your procrastination. It will challenge you to redefine yourself and to accept the fact that your tendency to procrastinate is a powerful force that you will have to learn to control. If you have made it this far in the book, you are ready for a new way of life. Keep up the good work.

# ⑨ "This Is Just How I Roll!"

**Directions:** START: Reassess your readiness for change.

→ Redefine your problem with procrastination.

→ Challenge your beliefs about yourself.

→ Figure out what kind of person you want to be.

END: Plan ahead so you don't lose your new direction.

You have made it through almost this entire book. That is a big accomplishment! By now either you have figured out why you procrastinate or you have some good clues about it. You have learned several different ways to break old habits, and you have started to change your ways. You should feel good about that.

You may recall from Chapter 1 that the Procrastinators Support Group recited the following pledge at the beginning of each meeting.

> *"I am a person who sometimes chooses to put things off for a while.*
>
> *"I usually have a good reason, even if I am not fully aware of it.*
>
> *"I have to admit that procrastination works for me some of the time, but I want to change.*
>
> *"I can learn to do things differently."*

Where do you stand now on each of these ideas? Are you ready to make lasting changes in your procrastination? This chapter focuses on going one more step in the direction of controlling your tendency to procrastinate. You have managed to get off your usual path and are headed in a more positive direction. Now you are at a crossroads. You can continue to be a procrastinator who works to control your behavior so you don't keep detouring off your chosen path, or you can try to make a more permanent change. If you want a more permanent solution, you must redefine yourself.

BOB: The meeting of the Procrastinators Support Group Chapter 121 is called to order. Donna, would you lead us in the pledge?

DONNA: OK, everybody. Here we go.

ALL: I am a person who sometimes chooses to put things off for a while.

I usually have a good reason, even if I am not fully aware of it.

I have to admit that procrastination works for me some of the time, but I want to change.

I can learn to do things differently.

BOB: Thank you, Donna.

LARRY (the new guy). I don't get it.

BOB: What don't you get?

LARRY: I'm not a procrastinator; I am a person who chooses to put things off. What's the difference?

DOROTHEA: There is a big difference. For a lot of us, procrastination has become a way of life. It has defined who we are, and we have spent years feeling inferior because of it.

ARTHUR: The difference in how we see it now is that procrastination is a thing we do, and sometimes we do it too much. It is an action. It does not define who we are. When we call ourselves procrastinators, it is like calling ourselves losers. If we think we are losers, we will act like losers.

BOB: When my procrastination had gotten so bad that I couldn't stand myself, I thought of myself not just as a procrastinator but as a weak and inadequate person. I was procrastinating on everything, even stupid little things. I had made it my lifestyle to put off until tomorrow everything that could be done today. It was ridiculous.

POLLY: We have worked together to redefine ourselves. When we stopped calling ourselves procrastinators like it defined us, we started to focus more on our actions and how to change them. It is better to think of ourselves as works in progress or people with potential.

DOROTHEA: I am a person with many traits. Sometimes I put things off to the last minute. I can change that. I *have* changed that.

LARRY: So I am just supposed to stop calling myself a procrastinator and that will fix everything?

ALL: No!

ARTHUR: It is only a start. When you change how you think about procrastination, it leads to all kinds of improvements. It makes you take responsibility instead of just saying "Oh well, I can't help it. I'm a procrastinator."

## Redefining Yourself

It may not be enough for you to make small changes in your behavior. If your procrastination affects many aspects of your life to a significant degree and has been a problem long enough for you to feel that it defines you, you may need a bigger and more powerful intervention. You may have to make the decision to be a different kind of person when it comes to taking action. You can begin by changing the label. Instead of being a procrastinator, it may be more helpful to say that you are a person who has trouble getting things done on time. When you say it that way, the solution seems obvious. You need strategies for getting things done on time. Try Changing Directions 23. The left column has a new way of describing the problem of procrastination. In the right column, write down an obvious solution to the problem. The first one was done for you.

---

↺ Changing Directions 23
## Reframe the Problem and Find a Solution

| I am not a procrastinator … | A possible solution might be to … |
| --- | --- |
| "I just have trouble getting things done on time." | Find a way to be on time. Schedule time for getting things done and put reminders on my calendar. |
| "I am just trying to cope." | |
| "I'm not sure this is a good idea." | |
| "I just don't like to be told what to do." | |
| "I just can't deal with stress." | |
| "I don't know where to start." | |
| "I've got too much to do." | |
| "I'm just tired." | |
| "I'd rather do something more fun." | |

---

"I get it," said Larry. "Instead of saying 'I'm just tired,' I should tell myself something like 'I'm tired right now, so I will rest for 15 minutes and then try again. And instead of saying 'I don't know where to start' and walking away, I should tell myself, 'Figure out where to start, and if you can't, ask for help.'"

"That's right," acknowledged Dorothea. "You have the idea."

"I know this stuff. It's common sense, but it doesn't seem to help," Larry said in a discouraged tone.

"Knowing and doing are two different things. Procrastinators usually know the right thing to do, the right thing to say, or the attitude that's best," Arthur explained. "You have to use your tools to figure out what is holding you back from using your common sense. Is it fear or self-doubt or control issues or disorganization or just plain old laziness? If you can figure out what is behind your procrastination, you can address the underlying problem. You are right that it is not enough to just tell yourself to get busy. If you procrastinate as often as the rest of us, you should start with asking yourself why you are procrastinating. If you can find your reason, you can find a way around it."

"That was great, Arthur," "You said it all," "Well said," "I agree," the group responded.

## Schema Change

When you redefine yourself, you don't just change the words you use to describe yourself; you change the music too. You alter your rhythm. You pick up the pace. Words are powerful agents of change. It is time to use them to reshape your self-view.

Schemas are beliefs that we hold not only about ourselves and our futures, but also about other people and the world in general. We pick up our schemas from our parents, siblings, teachers, friends, places of worship, and anywhere else that a message is given about how people should act or how the world should be. We learn from watching the important people in our lives. If they act like it is important to stay busy, then we learn that activity is important. We learn from the things our parents, grandparents, teachers, coaches, and other important adults say to us. If one of these people says, "You are a lazy bum, and nothing will ever become of you," we believe it. Our society, culture, community, peer groups, and families all shape our schemas by sending messages about how we should act, what we should think, and how we should feel.

Schemas are subjective. That means that two people can have the same experiences and develop two very different schemas. For example, if your mother had to work two jobs to pay the bills, you could have learned the value of hard work and sacrifice. Of course, some people would take away another message from such experiences. If Mom worked all the time and missed out on her children's activities, the children could have developed the schema that work is not more important than your children and you should never let money make you miss out on the important things in life.

There are schemas that can cause us to procrastinate and can keep us from making changes. Here are some examples of such schemas:

- "That's just the way I am, and I am never going to change."
- "If others don't like my procrastination, that is their problem."
- "I have been like this for so long that I don't know how else to be."
- "So what if I'm a procrastinator? The only one I hurt is me."

If you hold these ideas and are unwilling to bend, it will be hard for you to overcome your tendency to procrastinate. If you want to try to change your schemas about procrastination, try Changing Directions 24. With the help of the other group members, Larry worked through one of his schemas at the last Procrastinators Support Group meeting. His examples are provided after each step is described.

---

↻ Changing Directions 24
### How to Change Your Schemas about Procrastination

**Step 1: Identify your schema**. Pick a belief you have about procrastination that you think is keeping you from making improvements. You can use an example from the previous list or come up with one of your own.

---

Larry's schema: "I don't really think that people can change their ways."

---

**Step 2: What personal experiences have you had that suggest your schema is valid?** Make a list of events or experiences that are evidence that your schema is accurate.

---

Larry's evidence that his schema is true:

1. "I have tried to stop procrastinating in the past, and nothing has changed."
2. "I am 50 years old and set in my ways."
3. "I have been like this all of my life."

---

**Step 3: What personal experiences have you had that suggest your schema may not be accurate?** Include experiences that seemed contrary to or the opposite of your schema.

---

Larry's evidence that his schema might not always be true:

1. "I was able to quit smoking after 20 years of being a heavy smoker."
2. "When a lot is at stake, I can make important changes."
3. "My ex-wife said I would never change my eating habits, and she was wrong."

---

**Step 4: Weigh the evidence for and against your schema.** If there is reason to believe it is not completely true, perhaps it is time to change your belief. What would be a more accurate thing to say about your tendency to procrastinate?

---

Larry's new and more accurate schema:

"When I'm motivated, I can change. I'm motivated when the circumstances are important or when I have a good reason to stop procrastinating. It's all about the attitude."

---

**Step 5: In what ways does keeping your schema help you in your everyday life?** Think of the advantages of thinking that way. What does it do for you?

---

How the schema helps Larry:

1. "If I tell myself that change is not possible, I don't have to try."
2. "If I do make a change, everyone is happy. If I can't do it, no one is surprised. That way I don't look stupid."
3. "It gives me an excuse not to change."

---

**Step 6: In what ways does your current schema hurt you?**
What is the downside of continuing to think that way?

---

How the schema hurts Larry:

1. "I don't think it hurts me very much."
2. "I just stay the way I am."
3. "If I don't try, I can't fail."
4. "If I don't try, I will never get better."

---

**Step 7: Experiment with your schema.** If you think your schema is not entirely accurate and it hurts you in some situations, try changing it a little and see what happens. If you are still uncertain, try testing it out to see if it is always true.

---

Larry's plan: "I will try to change a little bit by not procrastinating on Mondays, Wednesdays, and Fridays. I will see how it goes. I know I can change, because I have already proven it in the past. I need to stop worrying about not being able to change and start focusing on gaining control over my procrastination."

Use this schema change exercise to help you rethink your negative assumptions about your ability to stop procrastinating. Larry had doubts about his ability to change. His willingness to be objective about this led him to a new solution. You may have called yourself a procrastinator for many years. It may have become part of your identity, who you are, and how you roll. It's time to think in a new direction. Read the next section on how to stop letting procrastination define you.

## When Your Procrastination Defines You

Does your procrastination speak for you? In Chapter 6, procrastination was described as a way of communicating your anger and need for control without having to say those words directly to another person. With anger and control, you make the decision of what you communicate to others through your procrastination. But what else might your procrastination be saying about you without your realizing it? Carla's delays gave her friend Melissa the impression that she didn't care about Melissa or her wedding plans. Bob's procrastination gave his ex-wife the impression that he did not wish to help her with the baby. Arthur's behavior suggested that he is not competent to do his job. Dorothea's procrastination made her father think she was not adjusting well to her new job or her new apartment.

What does your procrastination say about you? If you don't know, you should ask someone you trust to tell you the truth. If you don't like what you hear, it may be time to make some changes.

If your plan is to stop being a procrastinator, what will you be instead of that? Will you be the opposite of a procrastinator and never fall behind schedule? Will you allow procrastination to occur from time to time? Will you choose procrastination as a coping strategy when it seems like the right thing to do? There are many choices. Your challenge is to figure out how you want to change. Try Changing Directions 25. It may help you decide what you want to be.

---

↺ Changing Directions 25
### What Kind of Person Do You Want to Be?

If you're not going to be a procrastinator, what kind of person will you be? Try to fill in the blanks. It will help you begin to plan how you want to change.

---

Rather than avoid problems, I want to be the kind of person who _____
_____. (See Chapter 3)

When I get behind in my chores, I want to _____
_____. (See Chapter 4)

I don't want my lack of confidence to hold me back anymore. I want to _____
_____. (See Chapter 5)

I want to be the kind of person that other people _____
_____. (See Chapter 6)

If life becomes overwhelming, I want to be able to handle it by _____. (See Chapter 7)

I don't want people to think of me as lazy. I want them to think of me as _____
_____. (See Chapter 8)

Go back to the chapters listed at the end of each statement and review the Changing Directions exercises. They can help you become the person you want to be. While you are working toward making more lasting changes, use the following Shortcuts for redefining yourself to help you get a head start.

## ▶▶ Shortcuts for
## Redefining Yourself

Once you figure out what kind of person you want to be, you will have to find a way to get started in making those changes. One technique that therapists sometimes suggest is to try acting "as if" you are the person you want to be. It's similar to the "fake it until you make it" strategy. For example, if rather than avoid problems you want to be the kind of person who works on problems, asks for help, or resolves issues even when doing so feels uncomfortable, you should take some type of action as if that were the "real you." To get started, ask yourself something like "if I was not a procrastinator, what would be the first thing I would do to deal with the problem?" Another way to figure out your first step is to ask yourself what someone else would do to cope with the same problem without procrastinating. Take that first step and see how it feels. You might be a little unsteady at first trying to walk in someone else's shoes, but acting as if you were not a procrastinator is a good way to start heading in a better direction.

Arthur decided to try this strategy. Because it seemed like he procrastinated all the time, he decided that rather than waiting to catch himself procrastinating, he would just try to start his day off thinking like a nonprocrastinator. Arthur wasn't sure this strategy was going to work for him, so he thought of it as just an experiment. Experiments were like trial runs for Arthur. If the experiment failed, he would just alter the experiment and try it again, and he would not have to feel like a failure. The goal of his experiment was to procrastinate less this week than he had last week. To get himself started, Arthur put a note next to his alarm clock and on his bathroom mirror that read, "What would a nonprocrastinator do?"

On the first morning, he woke up to his alarm and was just about to hit the snooze button when the note caught his eye. He lay back down, closed his eyes for a few moments, and thought to himself, "What would a nonprocrastinator do right now?" The answer came quickly to him: "get out of bed." So he got out of bed instead of hitting the snooze alarm.

"Wow, that didn't seem so hard," he thought. He went into the kitchen to have a bowl of cereal. As he sat at the table he began to imagine what a nonprocrastinator would do next. He imagined a highly efficient person who jumped out of bed before dawn, put on his jogging shoes, ran five miles, and then returned home to make breakfast, clean the kitchen, do some paperwork like paying the bills, showered, and went off to work, whistling a happy tune the whole time. "I can't be like that," Arthur thought, feeling discouraged. Then he remembered the discussion they had had last week at the Procrastinators Support Group meeting about all-or-nothing procrastination. Don was like that. He did it all, or he did nothing. That wasn't like Arthur.

"If I'm not going to be a procrastinator, what am I going to do?" he wondered. Arthur needed a mental image of the ideal he was shooting for, a person who did not procrastinate as often as he did, but one who was not a binge worker or workaholic either. He thought of his sister, Allison, and how she seemed to be on top of things but did not overdo it. She procrastinated some of the time, but never to the degree that Arthur did, and she was not plagued with anxiety about how things would turn out, as Arthur was. That was how he wanted to be. He wanted to worry less and do more. That would be his mission. In the meantime, he was going to try to act as if he was not the type of procrastinator who avoided things. He would experiment with this one day at a time. He changed his note at home to "What would Allison do?" and put one on his desk that just read "Allison." He took a picture of her to work and placed it on his desk next to his computer. He had a clear picture in his mind of how his sister would handle most situations. So whenever he hesitated to take action, he could envision his sister being more proactive and tried to do what she would do.

Arthur didn't tell anyone in the support group what he was doing. Just in case his experiment failed, he did not want to be embarrassed by having to tell people about it. He decided that if he could go a full week acting as if he were not a procrastinator, he would consider telling the group.

At the end of the first week of acting like a nonprocrastinator, Arthur declared his experiment a success. He had procrastinated less often this week than last week. Rather than push himself any harder and set a higher goal, he decided that for the next week his experiment would be to try to stay at the same level and not backslide in his procrastination. He had read somewhere that it is better to take small steps at first when trying to change something important than to go for it all at once.

By the time the next meeting came around, Arthur had been

making small but important changes in his procrastination for nearly a month. Before he could tell the group about his progress, Olivia commented, "You seem different, Arthur. What's going on?"

"Nothing much," Arthur replied. "I just finally got around to getting a haircut."

"Looks nice," she complimented him. "New clothes too?"

"Yep. There was a sale this weekend, so I thought I should probably get a few new things for work."

"When was the last time you bought work clothes?" Olivia asked, knowing it had been at least two years since he last went to a shopping mall.

"It's been a while."

"Wow, Arthur, new clothes and a new haircut. You're looking good," noticed Claudia.

A little embarrassed by the attention, Arthur said meekly, "Thanks, Claudia."

Arthur was feeling pretty good about himself. He knew that his friends knew he had been procrastinating on getting a haircut since his old barber closed his shop a few months ago. And he knew that Olivia knew it had been several years since he had purchased any new clothing. He was grateful for their compliments and for their discretion in not making a big deal out of it. He had been trying to change in whatever way he could. He was far from overcoming his problem with procrastination on bigger issues, but he had hope that if he followed his sister's example, he might someday be able to say honestly that he was not a procrastinator.

## Making Changes That Last

Redefining who you are and how you approach tasks that you would rather avoid will take time, effort, and practice. It will not be enough that you have read through the exercises in this book and have a better understanding of your problem. You will need to practice the exercises, change your behaviors, and figure out what strategies work or do not work for you until it all becomes second nature. Change can be fragile at first. You might take two steps forward and one step backward as you try to change direction away from procrastination. To keep you from going in circles or back-tracking on your path to a new way of life, you will need four skills that will help you sustain your success:

1. Set reasonable goals.
2. Try to prevent relapses.
3. Accept your inner procrastinator.
4. Plan ahead for procrastination.

## Set Reasonable Goals

If your expectations are too high, you might accidentally set your-self up to fail. You will be more likely to succeed if you make it a practice to set goals that can be accomplished in the time you have available as was explained in Chapter 4. This is true for big life goals as well as smaller matters like finishing your chores. If you have forgotten, go back to Chapter 4 to refresh your memory on how to set realistic goals.

Another part of setting reasonable goals is time management. Chapter 4 also touched on time management skills. Time management begins with accurately assessing how much time you have available to get things done as well as estimating how much time a task will take. Procrastinators have a tendency to fool themselves into thinking they have plenty of time to get things done. If this is your problem, go back to Chapter 4 and reread the section called "Stop Fooling Your-self." If you set realistic goals, estimate your time accurately, and get a firm hold on your fantasies about meeting deadlines, you will be in a much better position to control your tendency to procrastinate.

## Try to Prevent Relapses

It is difficult to make big changes. It is even more difficult to keep yourself from falling back into old habits, especially during times of stress. Procrastination is one of your coping skills. Therefore, if in the future you find yourself overwhelmed, uncertain how to proceed, anxious, or exhausted, there is a good chance you will go back down that familiar road.

To prevent relapse, you must monitor your behavior. That includes keeping track of your tendency to procrastinate. One way to do this is to use the procrastination scale from Chapter 1. Review the items and check your procrastination severity score. If you are starting to revert to your old ways, perhaps it is time to review your notes and get back on the right track.

Relapses usually occur during times of stress and change. You will be at greatest risk of returning to your old ways during these times. If you anticipate big events like a job interview, moving to another city, having a child, or facing final exams, you can plan ahead to avoid procrastination.

Another way to prevent relapse is to address the emotions that make you want to procrastinate. If you have anxieties or fears like the ones described in Chapter 3, you can change directions using the exercises from that chapter to directly address your emotions rather than using avoidance as your way to cope. If anger is behind your procrastination, use the methods from Chapter 6 to communicate your feelings directly.

It may not be possible to avoid procrastination altogether, especially if you have relied on this way to cope for a long time. You can, however, learn to recover more quickly when relapses occur. If you are aware that you are slipping back into your old habits, you can put the brakes on and change directions. The overall goal is to avoid procrastination as often as possible. You may not want to give it up altogether. It is a coping tool that you can choose to use as it is needed and then put away.

## Accept Your Inner Procrastinator

Self-acceptance does not mean giving up. We all have weaknesses, and if yours is procrastination, it will do you some good to admit it and accept it. When you accept your weakness, you avoid the guilt that goes with being less than perfect. Procrastination no longer has to define you. It can be seen as a behavior pattern that shows itself from time to time. You can control your behavior. You can change. When you accept your inner procrastinator, you embrace the part of yourself that likes to be a little lazy at times, the pleasure seeker, and the inner child. It is OK to let your inner child out to play at times even if it causes a little procrastination. When you are ready, you can reel it back in and go back to acting like a grown-up.

## ᘒ *A Personal Note*

*My inner child likes to sleep late, especially on winter mornings when my bed is warm and cozy. My husband makes fun of me when I request "five more minutes" several times before having to get up and start the day. I know that of myself, and I accept that. Sometimes I decide procrastinating a little and lingering in bed a little longer than I should is worth it.*

*I admit that I sometimes use procrastination to regain control when someone is being overly demanding of my time. I probably use it as a tool to get others to step up and do their parts. I occasionally procrastinate on things that seem overwhelming or stressful or unpleasant. And there are times when I am just plain lazy and enjoy every minute of it. The trick is to live your life without the extremes of procrastination or compulsive workaholism. I get off track from time to time, recognize it, and readjust. I've learned that the kind of procrastination that leaves my mind stressed about what I should be doing instead is not a good kind of procrastination, so I have given it up. It's not worth it.*

*Now that I know what it is and I have control over it, I can use procrastination as a way of pacing myself so that I don't hit the wall after overdoing it with work. I still think that a little bit of procrastination is normal and can serve many purposes. If you are aware of what you are doing, you can gain control over it and use procrastination when you need it.*

If you have forgotten the difference between the good kind of laziness and procrastination, go back to Chapter 8. Follow the suggestions for getting the most out of your procrastination and enjoying those moments in life.

### Plan Ahead for Procrastination

Procrastination is a problem only if it is overdone. You get to decide how much procrastination to allow in your life. Rather than give it up altogether, you can set some limits on it. For example, I allow myself to procrastinate on exercise for three months out of every year. I know myself. I like to exercise, but I know there will be times when I am not in the mood, I would rather do something more enjoyable, or I just don't want to do it. I can have the unrealistic goal of exercising 12 months out of every year and feel guilty when I don't do it, or I can create a plan that works around my exercise procrastination. You can do the same.

Expecting yourself to give up procrastination altogether is like telling yourself that you have to be perfect. This is an unreasonable goal. Instead of expecting yourself to avoid procrastination all the time, make a plan to avoid it as often as possible. You can even decide that more procrastination is more allowable in one area, like washing your car, than it is in another, like washing your clothes. If you think you procrastinate more than half the time, you can decide that your goal is to procrastinate less than half the time. Just try to be reasonable with your goals.

# Procrastinators Support Group Chapter 121

The group has been meeting regularly for almost a year. Many of the members have reached their goals and moved on. New people have joined, and a few old-timers have stuck around to help coach them. Following is a brief update on each person you have read about. Most made changes in their procrastination. Some became more self-aware but have not made the move to change their actions. All felt less shame about their procrastination because they found others who had the same problem.

• Carla got her act together and helped Melissa with her wedding. She got a lecture from Melissa's mom about the stress she had caused others with her procrastination. It made a big impression on Carla.

• Larry proved himself wrong. He was able to make some changes with Arthur's help.

• Dorothea painted her walls and let her father paint the trim and doors. A month after she finally painted her living room, the building was sold and she had to move out.

• Polly made an effort to lower her perfectionistic standards when the situation didn't call for it. She even took a store-bought cake to a neighborhood party. Because she placed it on her own cake plate, no one knew the difference.

• Donna made a little bit of progress. She still procrastinates, but she doesn't feel bad about it anymore. When she has to scramble at the last minute to meet a deadline, she tells herself that it was worth it because she enjoyed her time off. Donna finally talked with her grandmother, who, as it turned out, already knew about Donna's divorce. She was warm and supportive.

• Arthur turned out to be a much better teacher than student. He helped lots of people overcome their tendencies to procrastinate, but still struggled with many of the meaningful changes he wanted to make in his life. He had used avoidance as his way to cope for so long that he was afraid to change. He got very good at recognizing the signs of too much procrastination in others. He started a second support group in the next town.

• Marta is still sensitive to being controlled by others, but she has learned to lighten up a bit with her new boyfriend. He had been in a controlling relationship and understood Marta's issues. When she becomes too intense, Mike can jokingly say, "Your inner control freak is coming out to play," and she calms down.

• Denise made a lot of progress. She gave up her habit of stalling until someone else took care of her problems. She wanted to have some control over her life, so, with Bob's and Carla's encouragement she overcame her self-doubt and began making good decisions. Things didn't always work out as she had planned, but she took comfort in knowing that she could make better decisions the next time.

• Terry is still a binge worker and wears herself out when she gets on a roll. She made a little bit of progress in pacing herself, so she procrastinates less often, but she still works with intensity once she gets going. Terry's periods of procrastination occur much less often and are more like times of rest than avoidance.

- Sally finally took a Spanish class.
- Claudia got the nerve and went to college. She is doing very well.
- My students waited until the last minute to write their term papers and still managed to do a good job. They all passed, and they still believe they do their best work under pressure.
- Olivia learned how to stop overcommitting. For a while she went in the opposite direction and refused to help anyone. After feeling like she could safely commit to helping out again, she began to take on new projects. The holiday season is Olivia's weakness. She still overcommits when it comes to helping at the local children's hospital, but it seems worth it to her.
- Bob made the most change of all the group members. He had not been a procrastinator until his marriage began to sour. Once he stopped being angry at his ex-wife, he was able to go back to his nonprocrastinating ways. He no longer goes to the group meetings, but he and Arthur stay in touch. When Arthur comes across a particularly bad case of procrastination, he calls on Bob to come by the group and share his story of success.
- As for me, I have not had time to procrastinate. I met my deadline for writing this book with one day to spare. My grant was submitted on time. I moved to my new house, and I decided it was OK to wait until spring break to finish unpacking my boxes. I plan to take a long vacation next summer and procrastinate for at least a month before classes start again.

The forces that make you procrastinate are still present. These forces include powerful ideas and feelings that can pull you off your path to progress and back on to the road to procrastination. If you want to change, you have to be strong. You have to believe in your ability to be better tomorrow than you were today. Remember the last line of the pledge: *"I can learn to do things differently."*

# Index

*Index*

# About the Author

**Monica Ramirez Basco, PhD**, is an internationally recognized expert in cognitive-behavioral therapy, a clinical psychologist, and a founding fellow of the Academy of Cognitive Therapy. She is on the Psychology faculty at the University of Texas at Arlington, with a secondary appointment in Psychiatry at the University of Texas Southwestern Medical Center at Dallas. Her books include the bestsellers *Never Good Enough* and *The Bipolar Workbook*.